HYPERTENSION

A Clinician's Guide to Diagnosis and Treatment

HYPERTENSION

A Clinician's Guide to Diagnosis and Treatment

BARRY J. SOBEL, M.D., FACP
Director
Encino Hypertension Center
Encino, California

GEORGE L. BAKRIS, M.D., FACP
Associate Professor of Preventive
and Internal Medicine
Director, Hypertension Training Program
Rush Medical College of Rush University
Chicago, Illinois

HANLEY & BELFUS, INC./ Philadelphia
MOSBY/ St. Louis • Baltimore • Boston • Carlsbad • Chicago • London
Madrid • Naples • New York • Philadelphia • Sydney • Tokyo • Toronto

Publisher: HANLEY & BELFUS, INC.
Medical Publishers
210 South 13th Street
Philadelphia, PA 19107
(215) 546-7293
FAX (215) 790-9330

North American and worldwide sales and distribution:

MOSBY
11830 Westline Industrial Drive
St. Louis, MO 63146

In Canada: Times Mirror Professional Publishing Ltd.
130 Flaska Drive
Markham, Ontario L6G 1B8
Canada

Library of Congress Cataloging-in-Publication Data

Hypertension : a clinician's guide to diagnosis and treatment / Barry J. Sobel, George L. Bakris.
p. cm.
Includes bibliographical references and index.
ISBN 1-56053-115-0
1. Hypertension—Outlines, syllabi, etc. I. Sobel, Barry J., 1951–
I. Bakris, George L., 1952– .
[DNLM: 1. Hypertension—diagnosis—outlines. 2. Hypertension—therapy—outlines. WG 18 H998 1994]
RC685.H8H7678 1994
616.1'32—dc20
DNLM/DLC
for Library of Congress 94-32780
CIP

HYPERTENSION: A CLINICIAN'S GUIDE TO DIAGNOSIS AND TREATMENT ISBN 1-56053-115-0

Library of Congress catalog card number 94-32780

Last digit is the print number: 9 8 7 6 5 4 3 2

DEDICATION

To our families

Contents

Preface

This book was developed for the busy clinician. It was designed to serve as a quick and up-to-date reference for physicians who evaluate and treat patients with *essential and secondary* hypertension. The manuscript was initially developed by one of the authors (BJS) to answer questions posed by clinicians at various symposia and lectures. With the aid of the coauthor, it subsequently grew into a book designed to meet the needs of clinicians who do not have time to look up specific clinical questions related to hypertension in encyclopedic textbooks.

This book is an accessible, quick and easy reference that makes available information on all facets of adult hypertension. Moreover, it provides references for detailed information about specific topics. The authors are grateful to the clinicians and academic nephrologists who reviewed and offered constructive criticisms of the text.

Barry J. Sobel, M.D., FACP
George L. Bakris, M.D., FACP

CHAPTER 1

Clinical Physiology and Pharmacology of Blood Pressure Control

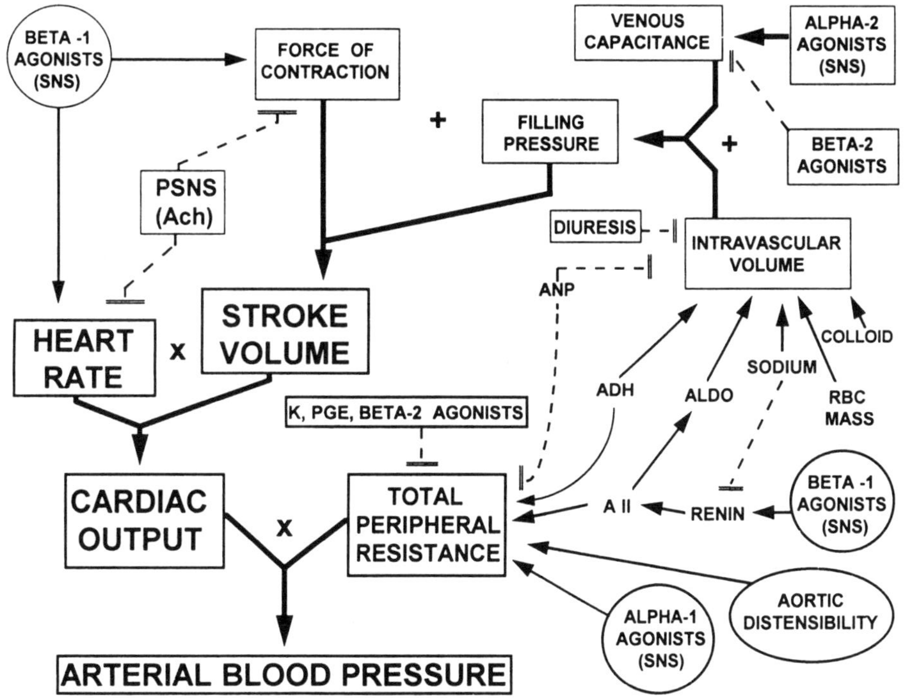

FIGURE 1. Factors responsible for arterial blood pressure. SNS = sympathetic nervous system; PNS = parasympathetic nervous system; Ach = acetylcholine; RBC = red blood cell; ADH = antidiuretic hormone; ALDO = aldosterone; ➔ = stimulatory (positive) influence; ---|| = inhibitory (negative) influence; A I = angiotensin I; A II = angiotensin II; ANP = atrial natriuretic peptide; K = potassium; PGE = prostaglandin E.

I. **Clinical physiology of hypertension: a clinician's outline**

A. Factors responsible for arterial blood pressure (Fig. 1)

1. Blood pressure is determined by **cardiac output** and **peripheral resistance**.
2. Cardiac output depends on **heart rate** and **stroke volume**.
   a. **Heart rate** is governed by:
      i. **Beta-1 receptors** stimulated by the sympathetic nerves.
      ii. **Cholinergic receptors** governed by the parasympathetic nerves.
   b. **Stroke volume** is determined by:
      i. **Force of contraction** (also influenced by the autonomic stimuli).
      ii. **Filling pressure** determined by:
         (a) **Venous capacitance**.
         (b) **Intravascular fluid volume**.
3. Both peripheral resistance and intravascular fluid volume are influenced by **neural, humoral,** and **renal** factors.
   a. Note that renal mechanisms are responsible for long-term maintenance of arterial pressure, whereas neural mechanisms are responsible for immediate (though less complete) regulation. When the arterial setpoint is abnormally high, it is the renal-fluid mechanism which maintains that level and prevents unlimited long-term increases in arterial pressure.

B. Feedback loops in the regulation of arterial blood pressure (Fig. 2)
Because of their number and complexity, no attempt is made here to cover all feedback and reflex mechanisms. Rather, an overview of the clinically most relevant ones is presented. For further information, the reader is referred to appropriate reviews listed at the end of this chapter.[1,5,8]

1. **Rapid responses and reflexes** (seconds)
   a. A **rise** in arterial blood pressure causes the baroreceptor system to respond by inhibiting sympathetic output and stimulating parasympathetic output (via the vagus nerve) from the central vasomotor center in the brainstem. This results in:
      i. Decreased sympathetic outflow to arterioles (decreasing peripheral resistance).
      ii. Decreased sympathetic outflow to veins (decreasing cardiac filling pressure).
      iii. Decreased sympathetic tone to the heart (slowing heart rate and reducing contractility).
      iv. Increased parasympathetic tone to the heart (slowing heart rate and reducing contractility).
      v. Little change in antidiuretic hormone (ADH) secretion:
         (a) Baroreceptors tonically inhibit ADH secretion normally.
         (b) During hypotension this tone decreases, leading to increased release of ADH (vasopressin).
         (c) In cases of severe hypotension, the vasoconstrictor action of ADH becomes important (and rapid).
         (d) The antidiuretic effect of ADH is a component of the slower-acting responses and is not important in the rapid feedback mechanisms (*see* below).
   b. Although several pathways are activated in the baroreceptor arc, each limb (represented in Figure 2 by separate connections via the vagus and sympathetic fibers) is capable of being activated separately under certain circumstances.

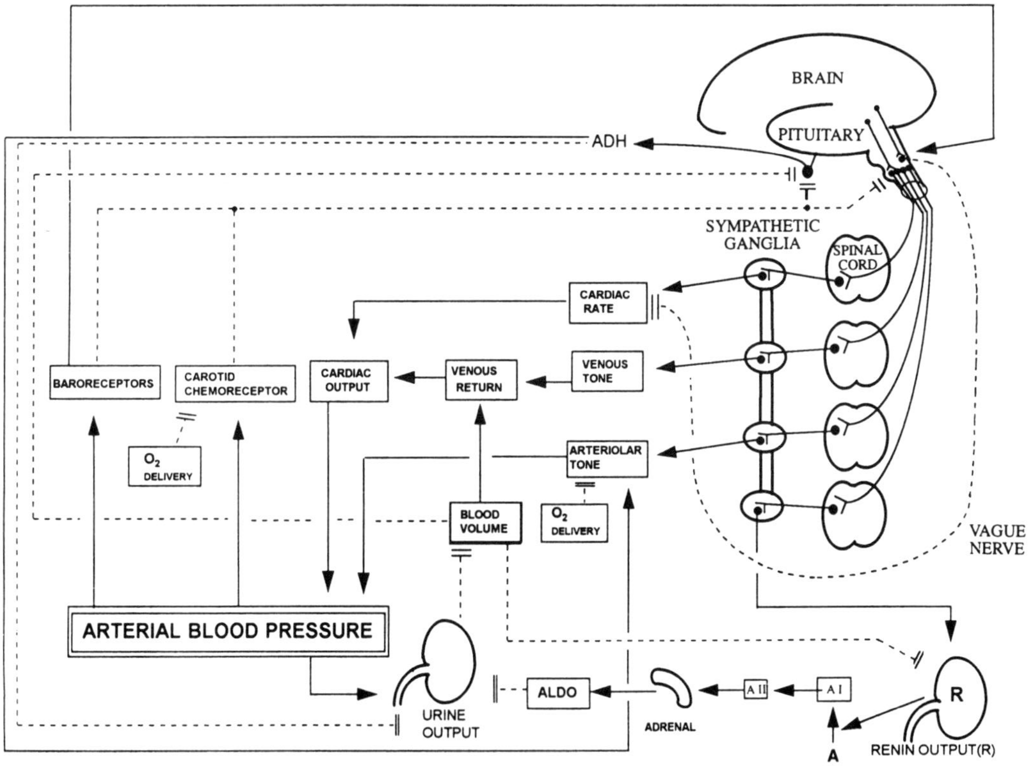

FIGURE 2. Feedback mechanisms in the control of blood pressure. ALDO = aldosterone; A = angiotensinogen; A I = angiotensin I; A II = angiotensin II; ADH = antidiuretic hormone; ➛ = stimulatory (positive) influence; ---|| = inhibitory (negative) influence.

c. **Chemoreceptors** also act at the vasomotor center but respond not only to arterial pressure but also to oxygen tension and carbon dioxide tension (in opposite directions). A **drop** in arterial pressure, a drop in oxygen tension, or a rise in carbon dioxide tension results in:
   i. Increased sympathetic outflow to skeletal arterioles.
   ii. Increased vagal tone, leading to slowing of heart rate.

d. The **central nervous system** (CNS, including supratentorial connections) itself senses ischemia or a rise in carbon dioxide in much the same way as the chemoreceptors do, and it can also influence the vasomotor center in various ways.

2. **Intermediate-acting responses** (minutes to hours)

a. **Renin-angiotensin system**
   i. Afferent arteriole baroreceptor causes renin release from the juxtaglomerular apparatus.
   ii. Macula densa mechanism
      (a) Renin secretion varies inversely with the chloride concentration reaching the thick ascending loop of Henle.[1]
   iii. Increased activity of the renal sympathetic nerves also increases renin release and often accompanies increased sympathetic outflow from other feedback loops.
   iv. Renin acts by converting angiotensinogen (synthesized in the liver) to angiotensin I.
   v. Angiotensin I is converted to angiotensin II by angiotensin-converting enzyme (ACE) (produced in the lungs).
   vi. Angiotensin II has two effects:
      (a) It is a potent vasoconstrictor (acting over minutes to hours).
      (b) It causes the adrenal gland to produce aldosterone over the next **several hours**; aldosterone action leads to volume expansion due to sodium retention.

b. **Antidiuretic hormone (ADH)**
   i. ADH secretion **increases in response to decreased blood volume** via a decrease in inhibitory tone from the **baroreceptors** to the hypothalamus.
   ii. A **rise in arterial pressure causes a decrease in secretion of ADH** related to increased baroreceptor activity, which normally inhibits hypothalamic ADH-releasing neurons.
   iii. Although increased secretion occurs in response to both increasing plasma osmolality and reduced intravascular volume, the response to rising osmolality is more immediate, while the response to reduced blood pressure (volume) is of greater magnitude.
   iv. ADH works by causing water conservation at the distal collecting duct of the nephron. This alone, without salt conservation, is a relatively inefficient mechanism of increasing intravascular volume, because water conserved is distributed among total body water and only a small portion of that is intravascular.

c. **Capillary filtration** (not shown)
   i. At higher arterial pressures, some fluid transudes across capillaries and into the interstitial space, reducing blood volume.

3. **Late-acting mechanisms** (days to weeks): Although these mechanisms take longer to activate, their long-term efficiency (gain) is greater than that with the shorter-acting systems.
   a. **Renal-body fluid system** (hours to days)
      i. A rise in arterial pressure leads to increased salt and water excretion directly (pressure diuresis).
      ii. ADH, in addition to acting as a pressor in the immediate response to severe hypotension and acting in the intermediate response to conserve blood volume, continues water conservation as long as the stimulus exists, and therefore is also a late-acting response as well.

C. Receptors mediating the control of blood pressure (Table 1)
   1. **Alpha-1 receptors**
      a. The peripheral postsynaptic receptor on the **arterioles:**
         i. Pressure is lowered by antagonism of this receptor.
   2. **Alpha-2 receptors**
      a. CNS synapse:
         i. **Stimulation is inhibitory** to the vasomotor output to arterioles, thereby **decreasing** peripheral neuron discharges and lowering peripheral resistance. Slowing of beta-1 output may also occur through the same mechanism at the heart.

TABLE 1. Receptors in the Modulation of Arterial Blood Pressure

Receptors	Agonist Actions	Agonists	Antagonists
Alpha-1	Vasoconstriction*	Norepinephrine >> dopamine > dolbutamine	Prazosin, labetalol
Alpha-2, central effect	Vasodilation	Clonidine, norepinephrine	
Alpha-2, peripheral effect	Venoconstriction	Clonidine, norepinephrine	
Alpha-1 and Alpha-2	Net vasoconstriction; reflex decreased cardiac output	Ergot, norepinephrine > epinephrine	Phentolamine, phenoxybenzamine
Beta-1	Increased cardiac output, lipolysis, increased renin	Epinephrine, norepinephrine, low-dose dopamine, dolbutamine†	Atenolol, metoprolol
Beta-2	Vasodilation,* bronchodilation	Albuterol, epinephrine >> norepinephrine	
Beta-1 and Beta-2	Net increased cardiac output	Epinephrine, isoproterenol	Propranolol, pindolol
Alpha-1 and Beta-1	Vasoconstriction and increased cardiac output	Epinephrine, high-dose dopamine	
Parasympathetic	Decreased cardiac output, decreased heart rate	Acetylcholine	Atropine

* Predominantly arteriolar.
† Without chronotropic effects (unlike dopamine and isoproterenol).

2. **Alpha-2 receptors** *(cont'd.)*
   b. Primary constrictor receptor on veins:
      i. Stimulation increases venous return.
      ii. The potential of increased venous return to cause increased cardiac output, and therefore higher pressure, is more than offset by arteriolar and cardiac effects due to baroreflexes in patients with an intact peripheral sympathetic nervous system.
3. **Beta-1 receptors**
   a. Heart:
      i. Stimulation results in increased heart rate.
      ii. Stimulation results in increased force of contraction.
   b. Kidney:
      i. Stimulation results in increased renin output.
4. **Beta-2 receptors**
   a. Arterioles: Stimulation results in relaxation.
   b. Bronchioles: Stimulation results in relaxation.

D. Neurotransmitters
1. **Epinephrine** (alpha-1, alpha-2 and beta-1, beta-2)
   a. Increase in heart rate
   b. No change or drop in blood pressure
2. **Norepinephrine** (alpha-1 and alpha-2 only)
   a. Hypertension without change in heart rate

E. Neurochemical interactions in the action of neuropharmacologic agents and blood vessel diameter (Fig. 3)
1. A blood pressure center within the brainstem is influenced by many forces, including baroreceptor feedback and supratentorial connections.
   a. Stimulation of central alpha-2 receptors inhibits alpha-1 and beta-1 output from the brainstem.
2. Neurons projecting from the brainstem synapse in the cord and those neurons, in turn, terminate in the sympathetic ganglia.
   a. Ganglionic blockers function at the sympathetic ganglia to block impulses there.
3. Electrical impulses cause the release of norepinephrine stored in granules.
   a. Guanethidine acts by replacing norepinephrine by incorporation into the granules, thereby depleting the stores of norepinephrine.
   b. Reserpine blocks the incorporation of neurotransmitter (norepinephrine) into granules.
4. After release from the presynaptic cell, norepinephrine attaches to the alpha receptors on the effector cells.
   a. Peripheral alpha-1 and nonselective alpha blockers prevent this.
5. After norepinephrine attaches to the effector alpha-1 receptor, a calcium channel activates the change in length of the muscle fibers.
   a. The uptake of calcium is blocked by calcium channel blockers.
6. Once norepinephrine reaches the extracellular cleft, it is removed by reuptake into the presynaptic cell and generalized metabolism via the blood stream.
   a. Reuptake is blocked by tricyclic antidepressants.
7. Norepinephrine also feeds back to alpha-2 receptors on the presynaptic nerve ending to lessen norepinephrine release.
   a. This action is blocked by nonspecific alpha blockers and alpha-2 blockers.

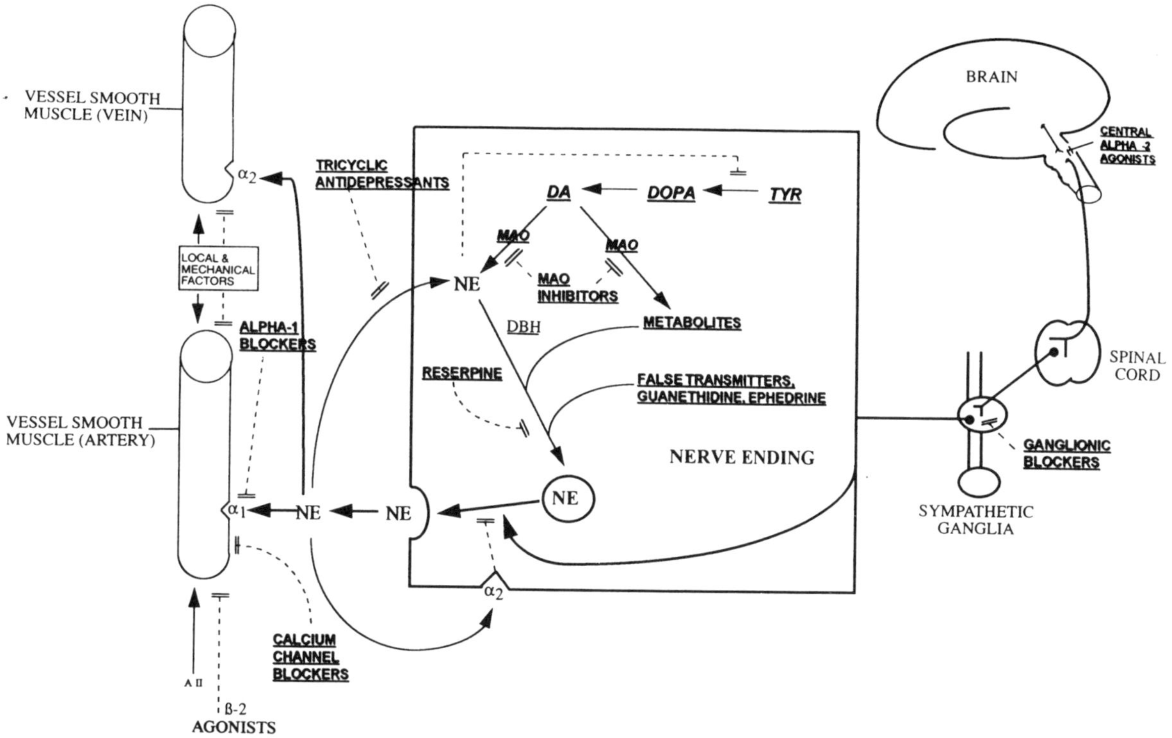

FIGURE 3. Neuropharmacologic interactions in the treatment of hypertension. A II = angiotensin II; NE = norepinephrine; TYR = tyrosine; DOPA = dihydroxyphenylalanine; DA = dopamine; MAO = monoamine oxidase; DBH = dopamine beta-hydroxylase; α_1 = α_1 receptors; α_2 = α_2 receptors; → = stimulatory (positive) influence; ---|| inhibitory (negative) influence.

II. **Mechanisms of antihypertensive drugs**

A. Central agents (alpha-2 agonists)

1. **Clonidine**
   a. Decreases sympathetic outflow to the beta-1 system receptors:
      i. Decreased cardiac output
      ii. Relative reduction in tendency of heart rate to rise
   b. Has little effect on alpha-1 receptor system:
      i. Baroreceptor reflexes are preserved.
      ii. Little change in peripheral resistance
   c. Acts directly on venous alpha-2 receptors to cause venoconstriction.
2. **Methyldopa**
   a. Decreases sympathetic outflow to the alpha-1 receptors of the arterioles, thereby reducing peripheral resistance with little (but some) effect on the heart. Some antinatriuretic effect occurs (probably due to some reduction in renal vascular resistance).
   b. Baroreceptor arc impaired because of action on arterioles.

B. Vasodilators

1. **"Direct" vasodilators** (hydralazine, diazoxide, minoxidil)
   a. Arteriolar effects only
   b. No direct cardiac effects; therefore, when used alone, direct vasodilators lead to reflex increases in heart rate and force of contraction.
   c. Require use of beta blockers and diuretics simultaneously in most cases.
2. **Calcium channel blockers**
   a. Arteriolar without venous dilation
   b. Relative impairment of cardiac conduction prevents reflex tachycardia.
   c. Have a slight natriuretic effect, and therefore total body sodium retention does not occur.
   d. Because arterioles are preferentially affected, transcapillary pressure increases, which may lead to local dependent edema, especially when cardiac output is not reduced.
   e. Drugs with greater cardiac depressant effects have lesser peripheral edema but a greater tendency toward increase in heart rate; drugs with less cardiodepressant effects lead to an increase in cardiac output and more peripheral edema.
3. **Alpha blockers**
   a. Nonselective
      i. Because they block both the postsynaptic receptor site *and* the presynaptic feedback site, catecholamine buildup within certain cells may lead to tachycardia due to release of catecholamines into the circulation with unopposed beta stimulation of the heart (tachycardia) and tachyphylaxis at other sites including the arterioles.
      ii. Nonselective inhibition of receptors in the gut leads to nausea, vomiting, and diarrhea.
   b. Selective alpha-1 blockers
      i. Block the action of norepinephrine at arteriolar receptors.
      ii. Selectivity prevents interference with feedback of norepinephrine and therefore no catecholamine buildup occurs.

C. Beta blockers
   1. Nonselective without instrinsic sympathomimetic activity (ISA)
      a. Central side effects (*see* Appendices V and VII)
      b. Antagonize sympathetic stimulation of renin secretion.
      c. Reduce cardiac output and heart rate.
   2. Beta "blockers" with ISA
      a. Intrinsic beta-1 agonist activity prevents direct cardiac effects.
      b. Noncardiac beta-2 stimulation leads to vasodilation.
      c. "Blockade" occurs mainly in response to stimuli.
   3. Beta-1 selective agents
      a. Have more effect on cardiac output and renin.
      b. Have less effect on peripheral resistance and bronchi.
   4. Beta-1-selective blockers with ISA
      a. Block beta-1 receptors at the heart and yet apparently have beta-2 agonist activity.

D. Diuretics
   1. Cause sodium loss.
   2. Cause some degree of vasodilation.
   3. Interestingly, calcium channel blockers also lead to net negative sodium balance.

E. Angiotensin-converting enzyme inhibitors
   1. Inhibit renin-mediated angiotensin II production.
   2. Have additional effects independent of the **systemic** renin-angiotensin axis, which are poorly understood but may include:
      a. Vasodilation dependent on increased levels of kinins because converting enzyme is also a kininase.[2]
      b. Vasodilation due to increase in certain prostaglandins.
   3. In patients with relatively low plasma renin levels, converting enzyme inhibition may work through the inhibition of **local** renin-angiotensin systems in vascular endothelium and possibly even the brain.[3,4]

REFERENCES

1. Lorenz JN, Greenberg SG, Briggs JP: The macula densa mechanism for control of renin secretion. Semin Nephrol 1993;13:531–542.
2. Williams GH: Converting enzyme inhibitors in the treatment of hypertension. N Engl J Med 1988;319:1517–1525.
3. Redgrave J, Rabinowe S, Hollenberg NK, Williams GH: Correction of abnormal renal blood flow response to angiotensin II by converting enzyme inhibition in essential hypertension. J Clin Invest 1985;75:1285–1290.
4. Johnston CI: Renin-angiotensin system: A dual tissue and hormonal system for cardiovascular control. J Hypertens 1992;10(suppl 7):S13.
5. Dustan HP: Pathophysiology of systemic hypertension. In Hurst JW, Schlant RC, Rackley CE, et al (eds): The Heart, Arteries and Veins, 7th ed. New York, McGraw Hill, 1990, pp 1140–1150.
6. Wallace AG: Pathophysiology of cardiovascular disease. In Smith LH, Thier SO (eds): Pathophysiology: The Biological Principles of Disease. Philadelphia, W.B. Saunders, 1981, pp 1122–1136.
7. Ferrario CM, Averill DB: Do primary dysfunctions in neural control of arterial blood pressure contribute to hypertension? Hypertension 1991;18(suppl I):I-38–I-51.
8. Guyton AC, Coleman AW, Cowley AW, et al: A systems approach to understanding long-range arterial blood pressure and hypertension. Circ Res 1974;35:159–176.

CHAPTER 2

Definitions, Epidemiology, Natural History, and Prognosis

I. **Types of hypertension**

A. Essential Hypertension

1. Defined as a persistent elevation of arterial pressure that results from a dysregulation of normal homeostatic control mechanisms in the absence of a detectable known secondary cause.
2. New definitions of **stages of hypertension** reflecting severity, according to Joint National Committee on Detection, Evaluation, and Treatment of High Blood Pressure (JNC V) guidelines,[1] are presented in Table 2.

TABLE 2. Stages of Hypertension (JNC V)*

Category		Systolic (mm Hg)*	**OR**	Diastolic (mm Hg)*
High normal (borderline)		130–139		85–89
Stage I	(mild)	140–159		90–99
Stage II	(moderate)	160–179		100–109
Stage III	(severe)	180–209		110–119
Stage IV	(very severe)	≥210		≥120

* The stage is defined by the **higher** of the systolic or diastolic.

B. Pseudohypertension

1. Readings taken with a blood pressure cuff reveal elevated readings that are not reflective of the true blood pressure measured directly by intra-arterial cannula.
2. Caused by relatively incompressible peripheral vessels due to calcific atherosclerosis.
3. Hypertensive end-organ damage is absent.
4. May be detected in some patients by Osler's maneuver (see physical examination, chapter 3).

C. Systolic hypertension

1. Proven benefit in treating:
   a. Mainly in stroke prevention[2]

D. Reactive hypertension

1. Secondary to an acute event:
   a. In many cases, studies indicate more harm than good may come from treatment:
      i. Drug withdrawal
      ii. Psychosis
      iii. Seizures
      iv. Stroke
   b. Treatment of reactive hypertension following stroke is **generally not recommended**, and no studies in animals or humans suggest that reactive hypertension following stroke should be treated.[3]
      i. Elevated blood pressure following stroke falls in patients given antihypertensives at a rate comparable to the rate it falls spontaneously.[4,5]
      ii. Patients treated do not have improvement in cerebral blood flow and may actually have a **decrease** in cerebral blood flow to the areas surrounding the infarction, causing an extension of infarct size.[6]
      iii. Serious complications of such treatment are reported.[7]

iv. Consensus favors withholding aggressive drug therapy.[3,8]
v. The level of elevation at which treatment should be considered (if any) is debated, since no data show that treating even very high pressures is beneficial.[3,4]
vi. In **subarachnoid hemorrhage**, nimodipine has shown value in reducing the cerebral vasospasm responsible for post-hemorrhagic ischemia, but treatment is ***not*** aimed at blood pressure control, and reversal of ischemia does not correlate with blood pressure reduction.[9–12] Reduction of blood pressure in such patients is potentially risky, especially if the patient has hydrocephalus, intracranial hemorrhage, or evidence of vasospasm.[3]

E. "White coat" hypertension and labile hypertension
   1. The patient's blood pressure is mainly elevated in the office ("white coat" hypertension) or alternates between normal and elevated (labile hypertension).
   2. Although this had been suspected to be a completely benign disorder, available data suggest risk may be intermediate between normal and persistent (sustained) hypertension.[13]
   3. Echocardiography may have a role in deciding if treatment is warranted.

F. Accelerated hypertension
   1. End-organ damage without papilledema or medical emergency
      a. Advancing renal insufficiency
      b. Funduscopic hemorrhages without papilledema

G. Malignant hypertension
   1. One or more of the following:
      a. Papilledema
      b. Pulmonary edema
      c. Neurologic findings (seizures, encephalopathy)
      d. Hypertension-induced angina

H. Secondary hypertension
   1. Defined as persistent hypertension due to a second underlying disorder other than essential hypertension. (*See* chapters 3 and 6, appendices I to IV.)

II. Basic statistics

A. Incidence
   1. Greater than 20% of the general adult population have hypertension.

B. Frequency of diagnosis (1991)
   1. 15% undiagnosed (15% of hypertensive patients have never had their blood pressure checked or, after having it checked, were not told of their elevated pressure.[1])

C. Medication compliance
   1. 50% incomplete compliance

D. Frequency of control
   1. Only 45% controlled (1988–91)[1]

E. Incidence by type (adults)
   1. Essential: 93–95%
   2. Renal: <3%
      a. Parenchymal: 2/3
      b. Renovascular: 1/3

3. Birth control pill usage: <3%
4. Primary aldosteronism: 0.3%
5. Cushing's syndrome: <0.1%
6. Pheochromocytoma: <0.1%
7. Miscellaneous: 0.2%

III. **Confounding variables in essential hypertension**
   A. Genetics
      1. Strong family history in most patients
   B. Environmental factors
      1. Salt sensitivity in about 60% of essential hypertension
      2. Obesity

IV. **Natural history and consequences**
   A. Increased risk of atherosclerosis
   B. If untreated, increases in severity
   C. Even if mild yet left untreated, leads to a high incidence of end-organ damage

V. **Prognosis**
   A. Treatment of even mild hypertension is associated with a decrease in the incidence of stroke.[14,15]
   B. Factors associated with higher morbidity and/or mortality
      1. African-Americans
      2. Youth onset
      3. Higher pressure
      4. Smoking
      5. Dyslipidemia
      6. Obesity
      7. Diabetes mellitus (doubles risk)
      8. Male gender
      9. Evidence of end-organ damage, especially left ventricular hypertrophy by electrocardiographic criteria
      10. Hyperinsulinemia (even without frank diabetes)
      11. Syndrome "X"
         a. Coronary artery disease
         b. Dyslipidemia
         c. Hypertension
         d. Hyperinsulinemia
         e. Hyperuricemia
   C. Stress and hypertension
      1. Stress may transiently elevate blood pressure.
      2. These elevations have ***not*** been shown to cause any morbidity or lead to sustained hypertension.[16]

REFERENCES

1. Gifford RD (chairman), et al: The fifth report of the Joint National Committee on Detection, Evaluation and Treatment of High Blood Pressure (JNC V). Arch Intern Med 1993;153–183.
2. SHEP Cooperative Research Group: Prevention of stroke by antihypertensive drug therapy. JAMA 1991;265:3256–3264.
3. Powers WJ: Acute hypertension after stroke: The scientific basis for treatment decisions. Neurology 1993;43:461–467.

4. Britton M, Carlson A, de Faire U: Blood pressure course with acute stroke and matched controls. Stroke 1986;17:861–864.
5. Lisk DR, Grotta JC, Lamki LM, et al: Should hypertension be treated after acute stroke? A randomized controlled trial using spectral photo emission computerized tomography. Arch Neurol 1993;50:855–862.
6. Meyer JS, Shimazu K, Fukuuchi Y, et al: Impaired neurogenic cerebrovascular control and dysautoregulation after stroke. Stroke 1973;4:169–186.
7. Britton M, de Faire U, Helmers C: Hazards of therapy for excessive hypertension in acute stroke. Acta Med Scand 1980;207:253–257.
8. Calhoun DA, Oparil SO: Treatment of hypertensive crisis. N Engl J Med 1990;323:1177–1183.
9. Allen GS, Ahn HS, Preziosi TJ, et al: Cerebral arterial spasm: A controlled trial of nimodipine in patients with subarachnoid hemorrhage. N Engl J Med 1983;308:619–624.
10. Petruk KC, West M, Mohr G, et al: Nimodipine treatment in poor grade aneurysm patients. J Neurosurg 1988;68:505–517.
11. Phillipon J, Grob R, Dagreou F, et al: Prevention of vasospasm in subarachnoid hemorrhage: A controlled study of nimodipine. Acta Neurochir (Wien) 1986;82:110–117.
12. Pickard JD, Murray GD, Illingworth R, et al: Effect of oral nimodipine on cerebral infarction and outcome after subarachnoid hemorrhage; British aneurysm nimodipine trial. BMJ 1989;298:636–642.
13. Cardillo C, De Felice F, Campia U, Folli G. Psychophysiological reactivity in white coat hypertension. Hypertension 1993;21:836–844.
14. Materson BJ, Reda JR, Cushman WJ, et al: Single drug therapy for hypertension in men: A comparison of six antihypertensive agents with placebo. N Engl J Med 1993;328:914–921.
15. Neaton JD, Grim RH Jr, Prineas RJ, et al: Treatment of mild hypertension study: Final results. JAMA 1993;270:713–724.
16. Freeman ZS: Stress and hypertension—A critical review. Med J Aust 1990;153:621–625.

CHAPTER 3

Evaluation of the Patient with Hypertension

I. **Purposes of evaluation**
   A. To uncover secondary causes of hypertension
   B. To establish a baseline and evaluate end-organ damage
   C. To determine additional risk factors
   D. To assess factors which may influence the type of treatment

II. **Understanding the causes of secondary hypertension**
   A. **Renal:** most common causes of secondary hypertension
      1. **Renal parenchymal diseases** (most common renal cause):
         a. Include:
            i. Glomerular diseases
               (a) Idiopathic
               (b) Secondary (e.g., diabetic nephropathy, lupus)
            ii. Tubulointerstitial diseases
               (a) Idiopathic
               (b) Secondary
            iii. Intrarenal vascular disease
               (a) Vasculitides
               (b) Scleroderma
         b. Hypertension is earlier and more frequent with glomerular and vascular conditions rather than tubulointerstitial diseases.
         c. Majority are volume (sodium)-dependent.
         d. Most important and most frequent cause of secondary hypertension in children and adults.
      2. **Renal artery stenosis**
         a. Major role of renin (at least in the absence of sodium repletion)
         b. Cure rate by angioplasty:
            i. 30% for nonostial atherosclerotic lesions
            ii. 90% for dysplasia
      3. **Obstruction**
         a. Very subtle at times
         b. Always a consideration, especially in
            i. Children
            ii. Diabetics
            iii. Elderly men
            iv. Labile hypertension
            v. Patients with recent pelvic surgery
   B. **Endocrine and metabolic**
      1. **Adrenal and adrenal-like entities**
         a. **Cushing's syndrome** (*see* Appendix I)
            i. Adrenal adenoma (or rarely carcinoma)
            ii. Hypothalamic/pituitary with adrenal hyperplasia
            iii. Ectopic ACTH secretion (especially from oat cell carcinoma)
            iv. Drugs
         b. **Primary hyperaldosteronism** (*see* Appendix II)
            i. High aldosterone *usually* with suppressed renin
            ii. Sodium dependent
            iii. Hypokalemia usually a hallmark
            iv. Types
               (a) **Adenoma**: curable, often unilateral
               (b) **Hyperplasia**: usually bilateral, incurable, more orthostatic, less hypokalemic

(c) **Glucocorticoid-suppressible hyperaldosteronism**[1]
(i) Usually **familial**
(ii) Onset usually before age 21 but can be adult
(iii) **Autosomal dominant**
(iv) Usually not spontaneously hypokalemic but become very hypokalemic with diuretics
(v) Elevated 18-hydroxycortisol and 18-oxocortisol

c. **Liddle's syndrome (rare)**[2–5]
i. Presents with hypertension and hypokalemic alkalosis, often with muscle weakness, polydipsia, polyuria, and (in children) growth retardation and failure to thrive.[6]
ii. Both plasma renin activity and aldosterone are suppressed.
iii. Responds to triamterene but not to spironolactone.

d. **Gordon's syndrome (rare)**[7]
i. Hyperkalemia with distal (type I) renal tubular acidosis and hypertension
ii. Clinical findings
(a) Short stature
(b) Muscle weakness
(c) Intellectual impairment
(d) Dental abnormalities
(e) Impaired growth during childhood
(f) Severe hypertension by third decade
iii. Laboratory findings
(a) Potassium typically over 6.5 mEq/L
(b) Acidosis with inappropriately high urine pH
(c) Suppressed renin and elevated aldosterone during hyperkalemia
(d) Serum aldosterone levels usually return toward normal after correction of serum potassium.
iv. Etiology thought to be a renal defect of sodium chloride hyperabsorption in the distal tubule
v. Dramatic improvement with salt restriction and/or thiazide diuretics

e. **Adrenogenital syndrome**
i. Hypertensive forms rarely present with onset in adulthood.
ii. Elevated deoxycorticosterone (DOC) with suppressed plasma renin activity
(a) 11-Hydroxylase deficiency—androgen excess
(b) 17-Hydroxylase deficiency—androgen and estrogen deficiency

f. **Pheochromocytoma**[8] (*see* Appendix III)
i. **50% have sustained (nonparoxysmal)** hypertension
ii. **Paroxysms of symptoms** often occur both in patients with and without paroxysmal hypertension:
(a) **Headache, sweating, and palpitations** are the three most frequent symptoms, though often not together.
iii. Other symptoms (in decreasing order of frequency):
(a) Pallor
(b) Nervousness
(c) Tremor
(d) Nausea

(e) Weakness
(f) Abdominal pain
(g) Dyspnea
(h) Dizziness, heat intolerance, and/or flushing

iv. Most common paroxysms involve **hypertension, sweating, and tachycardia**. Attacks are typically often brief and have acute onset (average attacks last 15 minutes).
v. Although the face may be flushed, the extremities are often pale.
vi. Precipitating factors which may provoke attacks:
(a) Smoking
(b) Induction of anesthesia
(c) Ganglionic blockers
(d) Hydralazine
(e) Massage of tumor, bending, or voiding (especially with large or bladder tumors)

vii. It is important to recognize that a patient may present with hyperglycemia due to this tumor and appear to have frequent "insulin reactions."
viii. Postural blood pressure drops are common.
ix. Hypermetabolic states may occur with or without coexisting hyperthyroidism.

2. **Juxtaglomerular tumor and ectopic hyperreninism**
   a. Very rare
   b. Present like hyperaldosteronism but with elevated plasma renin activity and normal renal arteries.
3. **Acromegaly**
   a. Hypertension, atherosclerosis, and cardiac hypertrophy associated with
      i. Typical features of the face and extremities
      ii. Sweating
      iii. Hypersomnolence
      iv. Weight gain
      v. Goiter
      vi. Carpal tunnel syndrome
      vii. Visual field changes
      viii. Hypertrichosis
      ix. Enlarged furrowed tongue, etc.
4. **Hypercalcemia**
   a. Particularly primary hyperparathyroidism
   b. May accompany pheochromocytoma
5. **Birth control pills**
   a. Associated with
      i. Age > 35
      ii. Family history of hypertension
      iii. Obesity
      iv. Higher estrogen dosage formulations
   b. Prognosis
      i. 50% resolve within 6 months after drug stopped.
6. **Thyroid**
   a. Hyperthyroidism: systolic hypertension
   b. Hypothyroidism: diastolic hypertension

C. **Coarctation of aorta**
1. Physical findings
   (*see* physical examination below)
2. Rib notching on chest x-ray

D. **Drugs**

TABLE 3. Drugs that Have Been Reported to Cause Hypertension

Birth control pills	Tobacco (especially in large amounts and/or with caffeine)
Licorice,[9] carbenoxalone, etc.*	Cyclosporine
Heavy metals	Chlorpromazine
Monoamine oxidase inhibitor plus tyramine, guanadrel, buspirone, or amantadine	Erythropoietin
	Depo-medroxyprogesterone[10]
Nonsteroidal anti-inflammatory drugs (NSAIDs)	Conjugated estrogens/diethylstilbestrol (DES)[11]
Sympathomimetics (including surreptitious)	Topical or inhaled fluorinated steroids[12,13]
Tricyclic antidepressants	Cocaine, amphetamines, etc.
Steroids	Alcohol

*Licorice contains a steroid (glycyrrhetinic acid) that inhibits 11-beta-hydroxysteroid dehydrogenase, leading to cortisol acting as the major endogenous mineralocorticoid because it is not metabolized to cortisone. Direct action of glycyrrhetinic acid is no longer thought to be the major cause of hypermineralocorticoidism in this syndrome.[9]

E. **Preeclampsia** (*see* chapter 6)

F. **Acute intermittent porphyria**
  1. May look like pheochromocytoma with
     a. Abdominal pain
     b. Back pain
     c. Muscle weakness with normal creatine phosphokinase (CPK)
     d. Postural hypotension
     e. Hyponatremia
     f. Fever
     g. Nausea and vomiting

G. **Other central nervous system disorders**
  1. Increased intracranial pressure
  2. Posterior fossa lesions
  3. Guillain-Barré syndrome
  4. Stroke
  5. Spinal cord lesions or spinal surgery

H. **Carotid sinus denervation (baroreceptor failure)**

III. **Approach to the patient[14]**

A. **History**
  1. **To detect secondary causes:**
     a. Age < 35 or > 55 favors secondary hypertension.
     b. Family history and past medical history
        i. Lack of family history may favor secondary hypertension.
        ii. Multiple endocrine neoplasia (MEN), von Hippel-Lindau syndrome, and neurofibromatosis are associated with pheochromocytoma.
        iii. Flank trauma or flank pain may point to renal ischemia.
        iv. Systolic hypertension may be due to
           (a) Severe anemia
           (b) Hyperthyroidism
           (c) Paget's disease of bone
           (d) Aortic insufficiency

c. Medication history (*see* Table 3)
   i. Including over the counter medications
      (a) Decongestants (e.g., nasal spray and cold remedies)
      (b) Antiasthmatic remedies (e.g., Primatene Mist)
      (c) Weight loss preparations
      (d) Nonsteroidal anti-inflammatory drugs
   ii. Herbal remedies
      (a) Herb teas used for weight loss
      (b) Other herbal preparations
d. Personal and social history
   i. Alcohol, particularly more than 1–2 drinks per day, may elevate arterial pressure.
   ii. Smoking
      (a) Particularly when combined with caffeine and or alcohol, smoking may exacerbate hypertension.
      (b) Nicotine in tobacco may exacerbate pheochromocytoma.
      (c) Most older patients with renovascular hypertension have a history of smoking.
   iii. Illicit drugs such as amphetamines and cocaine are important causes of hypertension.
   iv. Licorice-flavored foods, tobacco, and beverages
e. Review of systems
   i. Polyuria, polydipsia, or nocturia may suggest renal or endocrine disorders, especially in children.
   ii. Weight gain, ecchymoses, edema, new acne, change in libido or behavior, or change in menstrual patterns may point to Cushing's syndrome.
   iii. Oligomenorrhea and hirsutism may accompany Cushing's, thyroid, or adrenogenital syndromes.
   iv. Headache, diaphoresis, palpitations, postural hypotension, flushing, and heat intolerance may suggest pheochromocytoma.

2. **To assess end-organ status:**
   a. Angina or myocardial infarction (marked blood pressure reduction may be harmful)
   b. Transient cerebrovascular ischemic attacks (TIAs)
   c. Congestive heart failure
   d. Claudication
3. **To assess risk factors:**
   a. Tobacco
   b. Diabetes mellitus
   c. Family history of death due to vascular complications
   d. Lipid disorders

B. Physical examination
   1. **To detect secondary causes:**
      a. General
         i. Cushing's syndrome
            (a) Moon facies
            (b) Plethora
            (c) Ecchymoses
            (d) Truncal obesity
            (e) Purple striae

(f) Supraclavicular fullness (very common)
(g) Hirsutism

ii. Coarctation of the aorta:
(a) Unequal arm development or reduced development of lower extremities
(i) Very uncommon but much more specific than blood pressure inequality

iii. Marfanoid habitus in multiple endocrine neoplasia type III (2b)

iv. Hirsutism with or without genital virilism or infantilism may be a clue to adrenogenital syndromes.

v. Pallor of extremities (pheochromocytoma)

b. **Blood pressure**
i. Taken in both upper extremities, supine and standing, and in the leg if $<$ 35 years old
ii. In essential hypertension, diastolic rises upon standing; decrease suggests secondary hypertension.
iii. Unequal blood pressure in arms or leg pressure $\leq$ arm pressure
(a) More commonly due to atherosclerosis than coarctation
iv. Osler's maneuver
(a) Palpable brachial or radial artery with blood pressure cuff inflated above systolic to detect pseudohypertension
(b) Sensitivity controversial[15]

c. **Fundi:** retinal hemangiomas in von Hippel-Lindau syndrome

d. **Carotids:** bruits here suggest that atherosclerotic renal artery stenosis may be more likely.

e. **Extracardiac bruits**
i. In the chest may suggest coarctation.
ii. In the abdomen may suggest renal artery stenosis:
(a) Best heard lateral to the midline above the umbilicus or in the flanks.
(b) Systolic alone is not specific.
(c) Diastolic components are more specific.
(d) Bruits occur in 40% of patients with atherosclerotic renal artery stenosis.
iii. Cerebellar hemangioblastoma in von Hippel-Lindau syndrome

f. **Palpation of the abdomen**
i. Polycystic kidney disease
ii. Renal cysts of von Hippel-Lindau syndrome
iii. Rarely, vigorous palpation may cause a pheochromocytoma paroxysm.

g. **Café au lait spots**
i. Localized, flat areas of hyperpigmentation 0.5–12 cm in diameter.
ii. More than 5 spots over 1.5 cm in diameter suggests possible neurofibromatosis which is associated with both pheochromocytoma and renal artery fibromuscular dysplasia.

2. **To assess end organs:**
a. Fundi
b. Cardiac
c. Neurologic
d. Pulses and check for aneurysms
e. Edema, rales, jugular venous pressure

3. **Examination relevant to systolic hypertension:**
   a. Thyroid
   b. Tremor
   c. Pallor
   d. Aortic insufficiency

C. Basic initial laboratory evaluation
1. **Chemistry panel**
   a. Hypercalcemia
      i. Hyperparathyroidism
      ii. Multiple endocrine neoplasia
      iii. Pheochromocytoma
   b. Hyperglycemia
      i. Cushing's syndrome
      ii. Pheochromocytoma
      iii. Acromegaly
      iv. Coexistent primary diabetes mellitus
   c. Electrolyte abnormalities (*see* E.5 below)
2. Urinalysis
3. Electrocardiogram
4. Chest radiograph
5. Hematocrit
6. The absolute **minimum evaluation should include**
   a. Urine dipstick
   b. Hematocrit
   c. Potassium
   d. Creatinine
   e. Electrocardiogram

D. Additional laboratory tests
1. Echocardiogram
   a. Not routinely needed
   b. May be useful in making the decision to treat.
2. Home blood pressure monitoring
   a. Self-taken: especially useful in patients with negative family history and labile hypertension and those with apparent medication intolerance
   b. Ambulatory monitoring: useful in select cases (e.g., nocturnal syncope with no Holter monitor abnormalities)[16]
3. Renal ultrasound in all hypertensive children, those with symptoms of obstruction (including urinary frequency or polyuria), and those with elevated serum creatinines

E. Secondary hypertension: workup and "triggers" for further evaluation
1. **Onset at age < 25 or > 50** should suggest a workup for secondary hypertension, particularly:
   a. Renal parenchymal disease
   b. Renovascular hypertension
2. **Abdominal bruit:**
   a. Workup for renal artery stenosis if continuous (systolic and diastolic components both present)
   b. Isolated systolic bruit is not sufficient by itself to mandate a workup for renovascular hypertension.

TABLE 4. Causes of Labile and Resistant Hypertension

1. Dietary noncompliance
2. Drug noncompliance
3. Primary labile hypertension
4. Hyperthyroidism
5. Urinary retention or obstruction (even unilateral)[17]
6. Transient ischemic attacks, strokes, or cord lesions
7. Postural drop in blood pressure
8. Renal artery stenosis
9. Combined tobacco and caffeine (particularly in high doses)
10. Drug-related causes (see Table 5)
11. Pseudohypertension
12. Cardiac causes:
    Angina pectoris
    Myocardial infarction
    Aortic valve replacement
    Coronary bypass (pressor reflex)[18]
13. Office or "white coat" hypertension
14. Sleep apnea
15. Pheochromocytoma
16. Renal failure (volume or renin dependent)
17. Severe pain
18. Rapid drug inactivation (e.g., hydralazine + smoking, rifampin + propranolol)
19. Inappropriate combinations (e.g., methyldopa + beta blocker)
20. Alcohol or alcohol withdrawal
21. Malignant hypertension
22. Fluid retention reset syndrome (initially effective regimen fails in patient on adrenal inhibitor, vasodilator, or both; leads to compensatory intravascular volume expansion)
23. Wrong cuff size
24. Acute intermittent porphyria
25. Coarctation of aorta
26. Carcinoid syndrome
27. Acromegaly
28. Hyperaldosteronism
29. Scleroderma
30. Polyarteritis nodosa

3. **Resistant** (more difficult-to-control) hypertension without clear explanation: consider appropriate possibilities based on history and physical examination (Table 4).
4. **Postural hypotension**
   a. Pheochromocytoma
   b. Porphyria
   c. Renal artery stenosis
5. **Stigmata** or **classic history** leads to appropriate workup
   a. Moon facies, plethora, hyperglycemia, supraclavicular fullness, purple striae, edema, buffalo hump, truncal obesity: **Cushing's syndrome** (*see* Appendix I)
   b. Hypokalemia without other stigmata
      i. Hallmark of primary hyperaldosteronism (*see* Appendix II)
      ii. Common in renovascular hypertension
      iii. Additional clues to hyperaldosteronism:
         (a) Mild hypernatremia
         (b) Mild metabolic alkalosis
         (c) Hypomagnesemia
         (d) Lack of edema
      iv. Seen also in
         (a) Malignant hypertension
         (b) Cushing's syndrome
         (c) Liddle's syndrome*

* Liddle's syndrome is a condition simulating hypermineralocorticoidism with hypokalemic alkalosis and hypertension, but is a defect in the sodium-potassium exchange mechanism in the renal tubule, accompanied by suppression of both renin and aldosterone, without the presence of any abnormal steroid.

TABLE 5. Drug-related Causes of Labile and Resistant Hypertension

Nonsteroidal anti-inflammatory drugs (NSAIDs): antagonize all antihypertensives except perhaps central alpha agonists and calcium channel blockers.
Birth control pills
Steroids
Tricyclic antidepressants, especially with methyldopa or clonidine
Sympathomimetics, especially decongestants with beta blockers
Failure to use a diuretic, especially with volume-expanding antihypertensive medications
Inadequate dosage or inadequate frequency: e.g., once daily ACE inhibitor (breakthrough hypertension[19])
Use of a beta blocker in a patient withdrawn from clonidine[20]
Cyclosporine
Erythropoietin

v. Although adrenal hyperplasia can occur without hypokalemia, adenomas usually do not.

vi. Hypokalemia of mild severity (≥ 3.0 mEq/L)

(a) Not unusual in patients on diuretic therapy. Therefore, in patients **on diuretics**, a mildly depressed serum potassium alone is not grounds for further evaluation. (Significant hypokalemia in patients on diuretics is usually due to excessive salt intake or excessive diuretic dosage.)

(b) In the **absence of diuretic therapy** or another obvious cause, **even mild hypokalemia** should lead to consideration of secondary hypertension.

c. Palpitations, headaches, anxiety attacks, unusual sweating, hyperglycemia, weight loss; familial multiple endocrine neoplasia, or multiple café-au-lait spots: suspect **pheochromocytoma**.

d. Coarse facies, diaphoresis, acral enlargement, hypertrichosis, voice change, paresthesia, glucose intolerance, goiter, fibromata (many features similar to minoxidil side effects): **acromegaly**.

e. Episodic hypertension, back or abdominal pain, constipation, muscle weakness with normal CPK (paroxysms of hypertension last longer than in pheochromocytoma); fever, leukocytosis, postural hypotension, nausea, vomiting, sinus tachycardia, SIADH (syndrome of inappropriate antidiuretic hormone secretion), neuropathy: **acute intermittent porphyria**.

f. Consider **renal artery stenosis** workup (*see* Appendix IV) with

i. Age < 25 or > 50
ii. Young female (fibromuscular dysplasia)
iii. Severe hypertension
iv. Malignant hypertension
v. Continuous bruit
vi. Orthostatic drop in diastolic pressure
vii. Absence of family history of essential hypertension
viii. Neurofibromatosis

g. Urinary obstruction should be excluded in patients with hyperkalemia, polyuria, urinary frequency, nocturia, diabetes mellitus, or voiding difficulty

TABLE 6. Captopril Test Protocol*

1. Measure plasma renin activity and blood pressure sitting.	4. Criteria for a positive test (*all* must be satisfied):
2. Administer 50 mg of crushed captopril by mouth.	a. Stimulated renin of 10–12 μg/L/hr b. Increase in renin by 10 μg/L/hr c. Increase in renin by 150% or 400% if baseline < 3 μg/L/hr
3. Check plasma renin activity 1 hr later.	

* Avoid sodium restriction before the test.

TABLE 7. Captopril Renography[23,24]

1. Continue all usual medications except ACE inhibitors, which should be stopped 24 hr prior.	4. Do DTPA renography 1 hr later while replacing urinary losses.
2. Give 3 glasses of water at home.	5. Positive tests are *either* a. Peak activity ≥ 11 min b. GFR ratio > 1.5
3. Give 50 mg of crushed captopril by mouth.	

DTPA = ^{99m}diethylenetriaminepentaacetate; GFR = glomerular filtration rate.

6. Evaluation of patient suspected of having **renovascular hypertension**:
   a. To determine if **surgical correction** is indicated in hypertensive patients without azotemia, renal vein renin is no longer recommended since newer studies indicate it is not sufficiently accurate to be of value.[21] Clinical judgment is now used for deciding on the appropriateness of correction. Correction is indicated in azotemic individuals with renal artery stenosis to preserve renal function, regardless of whether or not they have renal artery stenosis–mediated hypertension.
   b. **"Screening tests"**
      i. **Direct arteriography (with digital subtraction if possible)** favored over screening tests in cases with high clinical suspicion without contraindication to the procedure (*see* Appendix IV).
      ii. **Captopril test** (Table 6)
         (a) Of limited utility by itself
         (b) Together with isotope renography, more useful but still not a completely reliable test
            (i) Not recommended as sole screening procedure
            (ii) Accuracy may be improved with sodium repletion and prior discontinuation of medications affecting the renin-angiotensin system directly (beta blockers, ACE inhibitors, and diuretics).[20]
      iii. **Captopril renography** (Table 7)
      iv. **Magnetic resonance angiography**
         (a) Good for main vessels
         (b) Not as good for nonmain arteries

REFERENCES

1. Rich GM, Ullick S, Cook S, et al: Glucocorticoid-remediable aldosteronism in a large kindred: Clinical spectrum and diagnosis using a characteristic biochemical prototype. Ann Intern Med 1992;116:813–820.

2. Wang C, Chan TK, Yeung RT, et al: The effect of triamterene and sodium intake on renin, aldosterone, and erythrocyte sodium transport in Liddle's syndrome. J Clin Endocrinol Metab 1981;52:1027–1032.
3. Mutoh S, Hirayama H, Ueda S, et al: Pseudohyperaldosteronism (Liddle's syndrome): A case report. J Urol 1986;135:557–558.
4. Nakada T, Koike H, Akiya T, et al: Liddle's syndrome, uncommon form of hyporeninemic hypoaldosteronism: Functional and histopathological studies. J Urol 1987;137: 636–640.
5. Takeuchi K, Abe K, Sato M, et al: Plasma aldosterone level in a female case of pseudohypoaldosteronism (Liddle's syndrome). Endocrinol Jpn 1989;36:167–173.
6. Fine RN: Clinical quiz. Pediatr Nephrol 1990;4:705–706.
7. Gordon RD: Syndrome of hypertension and hyperkalemia with normal glomerular filtration rate. Hypertension 1986;8:93.
8. DeQuatro V, Myers M, Campese VM: Pheochromocytoma: Diagnosis and therapy. In DeGroot LJ, Besser GM, Cahill GF, et al (eds): Endocrinology, 2nd ed. Philadelphia, W.B. Saunders, 1989, pp 1780–1800.
9. Farese RV, Biglieri EG, Shackleton CHL, et al: Licorice induced hypermineralocorticoidism. N Engl J Med 1991;325:1223–1227.
10. Leiman G: Depo-medroxyprogesterone as a contraceptive agent: Its effect on weight and blood pressure. Am J Obstet Gynecol 1972;114:97–102.
11. Crane MG, Harris JB: Estrogens and hypertension: Effect of discontinuing estrogens on blood pressure, exchangeable sodium and the renin-aldosterone system. Am J Med Sci 1978;276:33–55.
12. Vasconey F, Erez-Garcia R, et al: Hypermineralocorticism syndrome secondary to topical application of 9-alpha fluoroprednisolone. Med Clin (Barc) 1980;75:430.
13. Funder JW, Adam WR, Mantero F, et al: The etiology of a syndrome of factitious mineralocorticoid excess: A steroid-containing nasal spray. J Clin Endocrinol Metab 1979;49:842–846.
14. Slataper RM, Bakris GL: Secondary hypertension. In Taylor R (ed): Difficult Diagnosis II. Philadelphia, W.B. Saunders, 1992, pp 403–411.
15. Setaro JF, Black HR: Refractory hypertension. N Engl J Med 1993;27:543–547.
16. Grin JM, McCabe EJ, White WB: Management of hypertension after ambulatory blood pressure monitoring. Ann Intern Med 1993;118:833–837.
17. Weidmann P, Beretta-Piccoli C, Hirsh D, et al: Curable hypertension associated with unilateral hydronephrosis: Studies on the role of circulating renin. Ann Intern Med 1977;87:437–440.
18. Dustin HP, Tarazi RC: Cardiogenic hypertension. Annu Rev Med 1978;29:485–493.
19. Neutel JM, Smith DHG: Breakthrough hypertension. Cardiovasc 1991;12:38–40.
20. Bailey RR, Neale TJ: Rapid clonidine withdrawal and blood pressure overshoot exaggerated by beta-blockade. BMJ 1976:1:942–943.
21. Rudnick MR, Maxwell MH: Limitations of renin assays. In Narins RG (ed): Controversies in Nephrology and Hypertension. New York, Churchill-Livingstone, 1984, pp 123–160.
22. McCarthy JE, Weder AB: The captopril test and renovascular hypertension: A cautionary tale. Arch Intern Med 1990;150:493–495.
23. Setaro JF, Saddler MC, Chen CC, et al: Simplified captopril renography in diagnosis and treatment of renal artery stenosis. Hypertension. 1991;18:289–298.
24. Davidson R, Wilcox CS: Diagnostic usefulness of renal scanning after angiotensin converting enzyme inhibitors [editorial]. Hypertension 1991;18:299–303.
25. Black HR: Captopril renal scintography—A way to distinguish functional from anatomic renal artery stenosis. J Nucl Med 1992;33:2045–2046.

CHAPTER 4

Treatment of the Hypertensive Patient

I. **When to treat**

A. Anyone with a systolic pressure ≥ 140 mmHg and/or diastolic pressure ≥ 90 mmHg without a contraindication such as acute stroke[1] or postural hypotension should be treated.

B. Benefit in reduction of morbidity and mortality with mild hypertension is small but significant.[2]

C. Treatment of isolated systolic hypertension is beneficial.[4]

1. More likely to treat in patients with additional risk factors
2. A recent recommendation has been to treat patients whose systolic pressure consistently averaged 140 mmHg or more.[3]
3. Use drugs with very lowest risk of serious adverse reactions
   a. Avoid methyldopa, beta blockers, reserpine, ganglionic blockers, nifedipine).
   b. Consider low-dose clonidine, nitrates, very-low-dose diuretic with careful Na and K monitoring; cautious use of ACE inhibitors; or alpha-1 blocker with appropriate precautions.
4. Pseudohypertension must be excluded.
5. Orthostatic changes of dramatic degree preclude initiation of therapy and should be carefully watched for during therapy.[3]

D. Ambulatory blood pressure monitoring

1. Potential usefulness[4]
   a. Distinguishing "white coat" hypertension from sustained disease
   b. Confirming 24-hour control
   c. Studying significance of labile hypertension
   d. Studying nocturnal blood pressure
   e. Drug-resistant hypertension
   f. Hypotensive symptoms without apparent explanation
2. Has shown better correlation to end-organ damage than casual office readings so far.
3. Concerns that such technology would be overutilized have not been borne out by data.[5]
4. **Established norms**
   a. Mean of 135/85 mmHg in daytime but varies with age.[6]

E. Pressure goal

1. Generally 120–130/80–89 mmHg
2. It is unknown if further pressure reduction is beneficial.
3. Goal in isolated systolic hypertension is currently
   a. About 140 mmHg if BP initially is over 160 mmHg.
   b. 20 mmHg lower than initial if initial < 160 mmHg.

II. **Nondrug therapy (attempt in all patients)**

A. Stress reduction

1. Avoid unnecessary stress.
2. Rare cases require job change.
3. No evidence for long-term benefit of biofeedback

B. Diet

1. Moderate salt restriction = 2 gm sodium (5 gm NaCl)
   a. At least 50% of patients repond to this without drug therapy, at least partially (average 4 mmHg).
   b. Even in "nonresponders," it often markedly potentiates the effect of medications.

c. Assess compliance with 24-hour urine sodium (valid even if on diuretics, if they were started at least 3 weeks previously).
d. Greatest effect in older patients, African-Americans, and those with more severe hypertension

2. Higher calcium diet
   a. Controversial
   b. Most justifiable in patients at risk for osteoporosis
   c. May worsen calcium kidney stone disease.
3. Attainment of ideal body weight lowers blood pressure, even without salt restriction
4. Low-cholesterol, low-saturated-fat diet
5. Isotonic exercise within reason
6. Decreased ethanol intake
7. High-potassium diet (sufficient to maintain normal serum K; intake should be ≥ 60 mEq/day[8,9])
   a. Recommended in recent JNC-V recommendations
   b. Should *not* be recommended to any patient who is
      i. Hyperkalemic before therapy
      ii. On ACE inhibitors, potassium-sparing diuretics, or beta blockers
   c. May lower pressure further in patients on antihypertensives.[10]
8. Increasing celery intake (6–8 stalks per day) may reduce elevated arterial presures up to 20%.[10A,B]

C. Eliminate hypertension-worsening drugs (*see* Table 5):
   1. Nonsteroidal anti-inflammatory drugs (NSAIDs)
   2. Steroids
   3. Birth control pills
   4. Sympathomimetics
   5. Reduce tobacco use: reduces risk of coronary disease, stroke, subarachnoid hemorrhage, malignant hypertension, cancer, sudden death, and emphysema.

III. Drug Therapy (*see also* Appendix V)

A. Diuretics
   1. **Thiazides**
      a. Include
         i. Hydrochlorothiazide
         ii. Indapamide
         iii. Metolazone
      b. Generally effective and well tolerated
         i. Many patients cannot be adequately controlled without a diuretic; avoiding diuretics in such patients is clearly harmful.
      c. Drugs of choice for patients with recurrent **kidney stones** caused by hypercalciuria
      d. Dosage
         i. Should be initiated in very small doses (e.g., 12.5 mg hydrochlorothiazide daily).
         ii. Maximum dose 25 mg hydrochlorothiazide daily for control of hypertension:
            (a) At these lower doses, potassium levels below 3 are likely to be associated with noncompliance with salt restriction, or secondary hypertension (*see* potassium balance, below).

iii. Higher doses are more likely to be associated with adverse effects and *do not* lower blood pressure further in the majority of patients.
iv. Higher doses are often needed for treatment of hypercalciuria.
v. Higher doses associated with
(a) Hypokalemia
(b) Hyperlipidemia
(c) Hypomagnesemia
(d) Hyperuricemia
(e) Insulin resistance

e. Potassium balance:
i. As a rule, potassium is not affected in a clinically important way by small doses of diuretics currently recommended (unless the patient ingests a high salt diet, which will potentiate kaliuresis).
ii. Slight reduction of serum potassium need not be treated except[9–13]
(a) When symptomatic.
(b) When the patient is taking digitalis.
(c) With a history of arrhythmias.
(d) With a history of ischemic heart disease.
(e) With abnormal electrocardiogram.
(f) Prior to anesthesia.
(g) With liver disease.
(h) With carbohydrate intolerance (?).
iii. Significant hypokalemia while on diuretics may be a clue to
(a) Noncompliance with sodium restriction.
(b) Inadequate nutrition.
(c) Renal artery stenosis.
(d) Hypermineralocorticoidism.

f. Hyperlipidemia and diuretics
i. There is no evidence that long-term hyperlipidemia of any significance results from currently recommended doses of diuretics; indapamide does not seem to cause changes in serum lipids even transiently.

2. **Loop diuretics**
a. Include
i. Furosemide
ii. Bumetanide
iii. Ethacrynic acid
iv. Torsemide
b. Short duration of action mandates more frequent administration.
c. Many adverse effects more frequent than with thiazides
d. Generally required only with
i. Congestive heart failure
ii. Renal insufficiency, especially with concomitant vasodilator therapy

3. **Potassium-sparing diuretics**
a. Increased risk of hyperkalemia, especially
i. Without other diuretics
ii. With coadministration of ACE inhibitors
iii. With coadministration beta blockers

iv. With nonsteroidal anti-inflammatory drugs (NSAIDs)
v. With potassium administration
vi. In diabetes mellitus
vii. With renal diseases

b. Drugs available

i. Spironolactone
(a) Drug of choice in hyperaldosteronism
(b) Can be used to prevent potassium loss.

ii. Triamterene
(a) Also used to prevent hypokalemia
(b) No intrinsic antihypertensive activity
(c) Occasionally forms triamterene kidney stones.

iii. Amiloride
(a) May have a theoretical advantage over other potassium-sparing diuretics in diabetic patients.[16]
(b) Although usual maximal dose is 10 mg/d, doses up to 40 mg/d are often required when treating primary aldosteronism, and high doses of amiloride are usually better tolerated than high doses of spironolactone.

B. Adrenergic antagonists

1. **Agents active at alpha receptors**

a. **Central alpha-2 agonists:** inhibit central nervous system outflow to the preganglionic sympathetic fibers.

i. Clonidine
(a) Twice daily dosing is usually adequate.
(b) No orthostasis because although resting heart rate may fall, the baroreceptor reflex is preserved.
(c) Adjust the dose in renal insufficiency.
(d) Initiate dose of 0.1 mg nightly **once daily** in elderly patients.
(e) Severe rebound hypertension can occur if drug stopped suddenly.

ii. Methyldopa
(a) Twice to four-times daily dosing
(b) Orthostasis can occur because the primary vasomotor fibers affected control arteriolar tone, and therefore the baroreceptor reflex arc is impaired.

iii. Guanabenz
(a) Side effects less severe in some patients

iv. Guanfacine
(a) Similar to guanabenz

b. **Selective alpha-1 blockers**

i. Block norepinephrine action at the affected cell receptors.
ii. Have potential for first-dose orthostasis.
iii. Agents:
(a) Prazosin: relatively weak drug; requires twice or three-times daily dosing
(b) Terazosin: only one daily dose required
(c) Doxazosin: only one daily dose required
iv. Drugs of choice in patients with urinary retention due to prostatism

c. **Nonselective alpha blockers**
   i. Generally avoided in uncomplicated essential hypertension because of side effects and tolerance*
   ii. Useful in
      (a) Pheochromocytoma
      (b) Rebound hypertension
      (c) Monoamine oxidase inhibitor crises

2. **Postganglionic nerve ending-acting agents**
   a. Guanethidine and guanadrel
      i. Block norepinephrine release at the nerve ending.
      ii. Have greater effect on systolic pressure.
      iii. Orthostasis and gastrointestinal side effects make need for these drugs infrequent.
      iv. Are rarely used in the U.S. today.
   b. Reserpine
      i. Prevents norepinephrine storage.
      ii. Causes most of the side effects of guanethidine *plus* depression but less orthostasis and greater diastolic control.
      iii. Other newer, equally effective, and better tolerated drugs are now widely available.

3. **Beta blockers** (*see* Appendix V)
   a. Common to all beta blockers
      i. Sudden withdrawal may result in rebound hypertension, angina, or myocardial infarction, even in patients with no history of coronary disease.
      ii. Particularly useful for reversing secondary effects of other antihypertensives that limit the other drug's effectiveness, such as
         (a) Diuretics (which cause renin to increase)
         (b) Direct vasodilators (which cause tachycardia)
      iii. None of these drugs is safe for asthmatics with significant bronchospasm.
   b. **Nonselective beta blockers**
      i. Include propranolol, timolol, and nadolol.
   c. **Nonselective beta blockers with intrinsic sympathomimetic activity (ISA)**
      i. Include pindolol and levatol.
      ii. Are preferred for patients with symptomatic bradycardia.
      iii. Do not affect serum lipids.
      iv. May not be cardioprotective after myocardial infarction as other beta blockers are.
   d. **Selective beta-1 blockers (without ISA)**
      i. Include atenolol, metoprolol, and betaxolol.
      ii. May be slightly less likely to precipitate bronchospasm.
         (a) In practice, the selectivity is not complete and should not be depended upon in severe asthmatics.

---

*Because both presynaptic and postsynaptic receptors are blocked, the accumulation of norepinephrine at the synapse, which would feed back to stop further adrenergic output, does not take place. This leads to increasing norepinephrine release, leading in turn to escape from the antihypertensive action of the drug.

(b) This might make them a better choice in patients with chronic obstructive pulmonary disease **who require a beta blocker**, provided they have a history of mild or no bronchospasm.

iii. May also be a choice in diabetics who would benefit from their effects (e.g., post myocardial infarction).

(a) They are less likely to exacerbate hypertension during hypoglycemia and may not mask all of the symptoms of the condition **provided that they are given in low doses**, since these drugs lose selectivity at higher doses.

d. **Selective beta-1 blockers with ISA**

i. Include acebutolol.

ii. Like nonselective agents with ISA, may not be cardioprotective for patients post myocardial infarction.

C. **Direct vasodilators**

1. **Hydralazine**

a. Potent arterial vasodilator

b. No action on venous capacitance vessels

c. No postural changes (due to lack of action on venous capacitance vessels)

d. Compensatory tachycardia generally requires simultaneous use of beta blockers or central alpha-2 agonists.

e. Limiting the dose to 300 mg/day minimizes the chance of developing lupus-like syndrome.

2. **Minoxidil**

a. One of the most potent antihypertensives

b. Requires simultaneous use of **loop diuretic** and **beta blocker** or **central alpha agonist**.

c. Generally reserved for patients presenting with **accelerated or malignant hypertension**

d. Great utility in **resistant hypertension**

i. Virtually any hypertensive patient can be controlled with this drug when used as described, in combination with diuretic and adrenergic antagonist.

e. Hirsutism in most patients; females require use of depilatory.

f. Uncommon but serious risks of hemorrhagic pericarditis and tamponade

g. Rare cases of progressive pulmonary fibrosis

D. **Angiotensin-converting enzyme inhibitors (ACE inhibitors)**

1. Include

a. Captopril
b. Enalapril
c. Lisinopril
d. Ramipril
e. Benzapril
f. Fosinopril
g. Quinapril

2. Lowest overall side effect profile

3. Most common side effects and adverse reactions:

a. Profound hypotension when renin is activated:

i. Severe congestive heart failure

ii. Prior diuretic therapy

iii. Volume depletion or severe salt restriction

b. Azotemia when renal perfusion is renin-dependent:

i. Solitary kidney with renal artery stenosis

ii. Renal artery stenosis in kidney transplant

iii. Bilateral renal artery stenosis
iv. Azotemic patients without renal artery stenosis[17]

c. Life-threatening hyperkalemia: the more coexisting factors, the more likely the patient will become hyperkalemic:
i. Potassium supplements
ii. Diabetes mellitus
iii. Urinary obstruction
iv. Interstitial nephritis
v. Beta blockers
vi. Potassium-sparing diuretics
vii. Nonsteroidal anti-inflammatory drugs

d. Intractable cough: can occur with any ACE inhibitor.

4. Serious adverse effects (much less frequent)
a. Serious angioedema is probably the most common of the serious adverse reactions.
b. Agranulocytosis can occur with any ACE inhibitor (rarely).
c. Serious dermatologic complications (rarely)
d. Membranous nephropathy with nephrotic syndrome **at high doses**; very uncommon at doses employed currently

5. Effects in patients with diabetes mellitus
a. Attenuate the rise in microalbuminuria.[18–21]
b. Delay time to end-stage renal disease.[18–21]
c. Extra caution is required in diabetics.
i. If proteinuria worsens, consider other glomerular diseases.
ii. Hyperkalemia is commonly precipitated.
iii. Diabetics on these drugs **must** have at least two separate 24-hour urine protein determinations **before** and within the first 6 months during use of these drugs, or confusion is likely to arise when azotemia and/or more proteinuria occurs.

E. **Angiotensin II receptor antagonists**
1. Include
a. Losartan
2. Common adverse effects
a. Expect similar effects to ACE inhibitors in patients with azotemia, renal artery stenosis, congestive heart failure, etc.
b. Few nonrenal side effects
i. Cough: incidence same as placebo.
ii. Potassium: little reported hyperkalemia but **may still raise potassium levels.**
iii. Nasal congestion occurs in some patients.
iv. Rare serious allergic reactions and angioedema similar to those with ACE inhibitors have been reported.

F. **Calcium channel antagonists** (*see* Table 8)
1. Include
a. **Non-dihydropyridine calcium blockers**
i. Verapamil
(a) Most negatively inotropic
(b) Most constipating
(c) Least likely to cause orthostatic hypotension
(d) Least likely to cause peripheral edema
(e) Least likely to lead to tachycardia
ii. Diltiazem
(a) Intermediate in effects between dihydropyridine calcium blockers and verapamil

b. **Dihydropyridine calcium blockers**
   i. Nifedipine
      (a) Most severe orthostasis
      (b) Most severe edema
      (c) Most severe tachycardia
      (d) Most potent dihydropyridine
   ii. Amlodipine
   iii. Felodipine
   iv. Isradipine
   v. Bepridill

2. Major advantage is a lack of serious side effects in the vast majority of patients.
3. Usage is limited by constipation, especially in the elderly.
4. Annoying edema due to local effects, predominantly with dihydropyridine calcium channel blockers (nifedipine, felodipine), but may occur with any calcium channel blocker
   a. Due to a change in the transcapillary pressure in the extremities and should **not** be treated with increased diuresis
5. Potentially serious limiting side effects (Table 8)
   a. Dihydropyridines: orthostasis and tachycardia
   b. Diltiazem and verapamil: atrioventricular block
   c. All have some negative inotropic effect: verapamil > diltiazem > nifedipine/nicardipine
6. Less effective as second drug added to a diuretic

G. **Combined Alpha-1/Beta blocker with ISA**
   1. Labetalol
      a. Potent
      b. High incidence of postural hypotension
      c. Contraindications same as beta blockers
      d. Fatigue and impotence very common

IV. **Approach to therapy**

A. Customized therapy: Rather than simply using a "cookbook" approach, we favor an **individualized approach**,[22] when possible, to allow maximizing potential benefits and compliance while minimizing adverse reactions and side effects.
   1. **Noncompliant** or "no-show" **patient**
      a. Calcium blockers (once daily)
      b. Alpha-1 blockers
   2. **Post-myocardial infarction**
      a. Beta blockers without ISA have proven efficacy in lowering mortality.

TABLE 8. Comparison of Calcium Channel Blockers

Side Effects	Verapamil > Diltiazem	Dihydropyridines
Orthostasis	Less	More
Use with beta blockers or in the presence of atrioventricular block	No	Yes
Negative inotropic effects	More	Less
Tachycardia	Less	More
Constipation	More	Less
Edema	Less	More

   b. Heart rate-lowering calcium channel blockers (verapamil, diltiazem) have also shown efficacy in reducing mortality.[23–26]
   c. ACE inhibitors have been shown to improve outcome in patients with left ventricular dysfunction, even when that dysfunction is asymptomatic.[37]
3. **Anxiety or insomnia**
   a. Beta blockers
   b. Central alpha-2 agonists
4. **Renal impairment** (*see also* Appendix VI)
   a. Rigorous control of hypertension is critical to minimize progression of renal disease; analysis of data from a recent study of the effect of protein restriction on progression of renal disease revealed a dramatic effect of blood pressure control on delaying progression of renal disease (Fig. 4).[27,28]
   b. Goal of therapy is blood pressure of ≤ 130/80 if at all possible, which has been shown to delay deterioration of renal function, particularly in patients with over 1 gm/day of proteinuria. The effect is even more striking in black patients.[27,28]
   c. Effect of low-protein diets
      i. Modest protein restriction to 0.6 gm/kg/day seems to have some (relatively small) effect in slowing the progression of renal impairment; more severe restriction has shown little or no advantage. The recent Modification of Diet in Renal Disease (MDRD) study did show a much more dramatic effect of blood pressure reduction, which was far greater than the effect of diet.[27]
   d. Drugs of value
      i. Loop diuretics
      ii. Calcium channel blockers
      iii. Central agents
      iv. ACE inhibitors (only in low doses, or use fosinopril)
      v. ACE inhibitors with calcium channel blockers (preferred)[27]

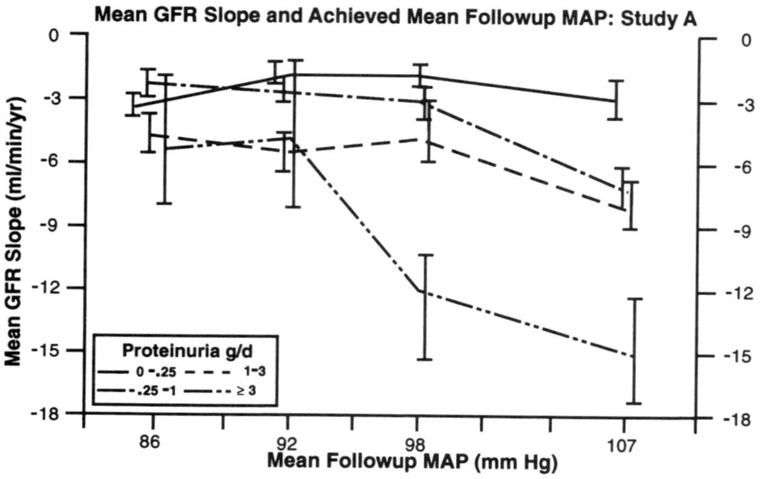

FIGURE 4. Mean glomerular filtration rate (GFR) slope and achieved mean follow-up arterial pressure.

5. **Migraine**
    a. Beta blockers
    b. Calcium channel blockers
    c. Central nervous system–acting agents
6. **Prostatic hypertrophy**
    a. Alpha-1 blockers
7. **Supraventricular tachycardias or angina**
    a. Beta blockers
    b. Heart rate-lowering calcium channel blockers
8. **Orthostasis or transient ischemic attacks**
    a. Clonidine
    b. Beta blockers
9. **Bradycardia**
    a. Direct vasodilators
10. **Left ventricular hypertrophy**[33,34]
    a. Nondihydropyridine calcium channel blockers[33,34]
    b. ACE inhibitors[32,33]
    c. Alpha blockers
    d. Beta blockers
    e. Central alpha agonists
    f. Diuretics[35]
11. **Congestive heart failure**
    a. Diuretics
    b. ACE inhibitors (cautiously, *avoid NSAIDs*)
        i. ACE inhibitors prolong survival in patients with CHF.[37–40]
    c. Angiotensin II antagonist
        i. Although preliminary results suggest losartan may be beneficial in this group,[40a] controlled long-term studies are not yet available.
12. **Essential tremor**
    a. Beta blockers
13. **Early diabetes mellitus** (microalbuminuria with no azotemia)
    a. ACE inhibitors alone (with careful monitoring of potassium) preferred.
        i. In **type I** diabetes, this treatment has been shown to slow progression of **both**
            (a) Established renal disease[41] **and**
            (b) Microalbuminuria in patients without azotemia.
        ii. As noted in a recent editorial,[42] this treatment slows deterioration of renal function in **both normotensive type I**[43] **and normotensive type II**[44] patients **with microalbuminuria and initially normal renal function.**
    b. ACE inhibitors with calcium channel blockers added: only for coronary disease or difficult-to-control hypertension; nondihydropyridine types preferred.*[22,23,45]
    c. ACE inhibitors with diuretics: for difficult-to-control hypertension with sodium retention due to
        i. Congestive heart failure
        ii. Edema due to renal failure or nephrotic syndrome

---

*Although addition of nondihydropyridine calcium channel blockers to angiotensin-converting inhibitors further reduces proteinuria, it is currently unknown whether this has a beneficial long-term effect on human renal function; a recent animal study showed that ACE inhibitors or the combination of ACE inhibitors and nondihydropyridine calcium blockers prevented mesangial expansion.[45]

d. Alpha blockers also can be used without adverse effects but have not been shown to have the potential benefits of the other regimens on preservation of renal function.
e. When beta blockers are required, beta-1 selective agents in the lowest possible doses should be used.
    i. There is no evidence that these drugs have the renal benefits of other drugs (such as ACE inhibitors).
    ii. Addition will make hyperkalemia more likely.
    iii. Sometimes required (e.g., post-myocardial infarction and angina unresponsive to calcium channel blockers alone)

14. **Late diabetes mellitus** (serum creatinine $\geq$ 1.5 mg/dl and proteinuria over 1 gm/24 hr)
    a. Diuretics almost always required
    b. Calcium channel blockers, with or without ACE inhibitors, in reduced dosage:
        i. There is evidence that once proteinuria or azotemia is established, ACE inhibitors may still slow progression of renal disease.
        ii. Close monitoring of creatinine and potassium as well as the magnitude of proteinuria is required.
        iii. Recent data suggest that antihypertensive agents that blunt the rise in proteinuria over time preserve renal function to a greater extent than agents that do not have these effects.[21–23,26,27] This may apply even in the absence of changes in blood pressure.[19] These agents are primarily the ACE inhibitors and nondihydropyridine calcium channel blockers.
    c. One recent study suggested that in **azotemic patients with frank proteinuria**, a low-protein, low-phosphorus diet might delay progression of diabetic nephropathy.[46]
15. **Accelerated or malignant hypertension**
    a. ACE inhibitors
    b. Minoxidil or hydralazine (with diuretics and beta blockers)
16. **Young patients**
    a. ACE inhibitors (except avoid in women who may become pregnant)
    b. Calcium blockers
    c. Alpha-1 blockers
17. **Young and "hyperdynamic" persons**
    a. Verapamil
    b. Beta blockers without ISA
18. **Isolated systolic hypertension**
    a. Diuretics[1]
    b. Long-acting isosorbide[47]
    c. Calcium channel blockers
    d. Low-dose labetalol[48]
19. **Elderly patients**
    a. Diuretics
    b. Calcium blockers
    c. ACE inhibitors
    d. Nitrates (with systolic hypertension, especially with history of coronary artery disease)

20. **African-Americans** (especially young)
    a. Diuretics
    b. Calcium blockers
    c. Labetalol (monitor liver function tests, stop drug if abnormal)
    d. ACE inhibitors in moderate to high doses
21. **Obesity**
    a. Diuretics
    b. Calcium blockers
22. **Young women intending to have children**
    a. Avoid ACE inhibitors.
    b. Methyldopa (preferred)
    c. Atenolol, metoprolol
23. **Hyperlipidemia**
    a. Alpha blockers
    b. Calcium blockers
    c. ACE inhibitors
    d. Indapamide
    e. Beta blockers with ISA
24. **Renal artery stenosis**
    a. Calcium channel blockers
    b. Beta blockers
    c. Minoxidil in resistant cases
    d. Avoid ACE inhibitors in cases with bilateral disease, solitary kidney, stenosis to a renal transplant, and unilateral stenosis with significant azotemia (significant nephrosclerosis).
25. **Nephrolithiasis due to hypercalciuria** (most kidney stones)
    a. Thiazides
26. **Post-renal transplant**
    a. Calcium blockers
        i. With dihydropyridines, generally no cyclosporine dose adjustment is needed.
        ii. With verapamil and diltiazem, cyclosporine dose must be reduced.
    b. Central agents
    c. Labetalol
27. **Arthritis** (33% of hypertensive patients)
    a. Calcium blockers
    b. Alpha blockers
    c. Avoid ACE inhibitors if on NSAIDs.
        i. The nonacetylated (non-aspirinlike) salicylates, such as salsalate (Disalcid) and choline magnesium trisalicylate (Trilisate), may be the least likely to interact with antihypertensive medications.
        ii. Among traditional NSAIDs, sulindac (Clinoril) seems to interact least often; naproxen may also be less likely to interact. Most others antagonize anithypertensives.
    d. Coadministration of potassium-sparing diuretics and beta blockers, as well as ACE inhibitors, will result in a higher incidence of hyperkalemia with NSAIDs. Close monitoring of potassium and creatinine is mandatory when any of these is combined with an NSAID. Generally, use of potassium-sparing diuretics with an ACE inhibitor is contraindicated.

28. **Liver disease**
    a. With portal hypertension, consider nonselective beta blockers.
    b. Avoid labetalol, methyldopa, and ACE inhibitors (especially NSAIDs).
    c. Avoid methyldopa.
29. **Asthma and chronic obstructive pulmonary disease (COPD)**
    a. Calcium channel blockers are preferred (especially dihydropyridines).[49,50]
    b. Beta blockers of all types are contraindicated, except beta-1 selective agents may be used **cautiously if necessary** and in **low doses** in patients who have COPD but **no history of bronchospasm**.
    c. Use of the following is possible in low doses and with caution:
        i. Central alpha-2 agonists and alpha-1 blockers: May increase subjective dyspnea or increase sensitivity to histamine.[51,52]
        ii. Diuretics
            (a) Hypokalemia will be additive to that induced by inhaled or oral beta agonists and steroids.
            (b) Metabolic alkalosis may reduce hypoxic drive in patients with severe COPD.
            (c) In patients on theophylline preparations, the tendency to arrhythmias and seizures is likely to be enhanced by hypokalemia or alkalosis.
        iii. ACE inhibitors (avoid if possible): may increase histamine release and precipitate asthma in such individuals.[53]
30. **Pheochromocytoma**[54] (*see* Appendix III for perioperative management)
    a. Medical management is necessary until surgery and during pregnancy. It is also required in patients with metastatic malignant pheochromocytoma.
    b. Drug therapy
        i. Nonselective alpha blockers have been the mainstay of therapy:
            (a) Phenoxybenzamine, 10–20 mg four times daily and titrated to control pressure.
        ii. Peripheral alpha-2 blockers, such as prazosin, also have been used.
        iii. Calcium channel blockers also have been used effectively and have the theoretical advantages of avoiding postural hypotension and overshoot hypotension.
        iv. Beta blockers may be needed in patients with disproportionate beta-1 (epinephrine-like) activity; however, this is **contraindicated** until the patient is well alpha-blocked, since beta-2 activity produces vasodilation and antagonizes vasoconstrictive alpha-1 effects. If beta blockade alone is used, hypertension may dramatically worsen.
        v. During surgery:
            (a) Nitroprusside and/or phentolamine are used parenterally.
            (b) The short-acting beta blocker esmolol may be **added**, if necessary, to control cardiac arrhythmias, although lidocaine also has been used.

31. **Hyperaldosteronism**[44]
    a. Solitary tumors are usually resected.
    b. Drug therapy
        i. In adrenal hyperplasia, spironolactone is the drug of choice (up to 400 mg/day).
        ii. Amiloride (up to 40 mg/d) may be used in place of spironolactone to lessen side effects, particularly in men.
        iii. Triamterene is not as effective but may be tried in patients intolerant of spironolactone and amiloride.
        iv. In many cases, thiazide diuretics need to be added (12.5–25 mg hydrochlorothiazide daily).
        v. Some patients may need the addition of a third drug: calcium blockers and ACE inhibitors have been suggested as effective options.
    c. In all cases, careful monitoring of serum potassium during therapy is needed.
    d. Postoperative **hypo**aldosteronism may occur and so **potassium must be monitored after surgery**; during that time, potassium should be administered only with great caution.
32. **Adrenogenital syndrome** and **glucocorticoid-responsive hyperaldosteronism** (*see* Appendix II)
    a. Treat with low-dose prednisone (e.g., 5–7 mg/day).
    b. Occasional patients may require slightly higher doses.
    c. Patients require increased doses during stress.

B. Without coexisting diseases or conditions listed above (Fig. 5)
C. Be aware of potential side side effects (*see* Appendix VII).
1. Sensitivity by the physician to benign yet annoying side effects will increase compliance.
2. Monitor appropriate parameters when using drugs with potentially serious side effects:
    a. **Potassium**
        i. ACE inhibitors
        ii. Diuretics
        iii. Beta blockers (if diabetic or azotemic)
    b. **Liver function**
        i. Labetalol
        ii. Methyldopa
        iii. Hydralazine
    c. **Blood counts**
        i. ACE inhibitors
        ii. Methyldopa
        iii. Hydralazine
        iv. Diuretics
        v. Minoxidil
    d. **Renal function** should be monitored in all hypertensive patients but is particularly important in:
        i. All diabetics
        ii. All patients on beta blockers
        iii. All patients on ACE inhibitors
        iv. All patients on diuretics

Salt restriction (2 gm Na = 80 mEq Na), weight loss, exercise, reduction of tobacco, reduction of alcohol

↓ Pressure remains elevated

Start low-dose thiazide, beta blocker, calcium blocker, low-dose ACE inhibitor, or peripheral alpha-1 blocker

↓ Pressure remains elevated

Double initial dosage

↓ Pressure remains elevated

Add a low-dose thiazide or substitute another drug

↓ Pressure remains elevated

Full dose current drug

↓ Pressure remains elevated

Reevaluate:
- Compliance with diet or medications
- Secondary causes
- Intraarterial blood pressure especially in the elderly[55]
- Ambulatory blood pressure monitoring

↓ Pressure remains elevated

Add ACE inhibitor if not already being used (caution if on diuretic)

↓ Pressure remains elevated

Add calcium antagonist if not already being used

↓ Pressure remains elevated

Add appropriate drug from another class, such as
- Clonidine
- Hydralazine
- Beta blockers (caution with calcium blockers)

↓ Pressure remains elevated

Add minoxidil, withdraw all medications, except beta blocker or clonidine, and loop diuretic

↓ Pressure remains elevated

Strongly consider either noncompliance or secondary cause

FIGURE 5. An approach to blood pressure reduction in the uncomplicated hypertensive patient.

REFERENCES

1. Powers WJ: Acute hypertension after stroke: The scientific basis for treatment decisions. Neurology 1993;43;461–467.
2. SHEP Cooperative Research Group: Prevention of stroke by antihypertensive drug treatment in older persons with isolated systolic hypertension. JAMA 1991;265:3255–3264.
3. Michelis MF: Systolic hypertension in the elderly: Reasons not to treat. Am J Kid Dis 1990;16:332–334.
4. Gifford RW, Chairman, et al: The fifth report of the Joint National Committee on Detection, Evaluation, and Treatment of High Blood Pressure (JNC V). Arch Intern Med 1993;153:154–183.
5. Grin JM, McCabe EJ, White WB: Management of hypertension after ambulatory blood pressure monitoring. Ann Intern Med 1993;118:833–837.
6. Zachariah PK, Sheps SG, Bailey KR, et al: Age-related characteristics of ambulatory blood pressure load and mean blood pressure in normal subjects. JAMA 1991;265:1414–1417.
7. Reference deleted.
8. Linas SL: The role of potassium in the pathogenesis of hypertension. Kidney Int 1991;39:771–786.
9. Khaw KT, Barrett-Conner E: Dietary potassium and stroke-related mortality: A 12-year prospective population study. N Engl J Med 1987;316:236–240.
10. Siani A, Strazzullo P, Giacco A, et al: Increasing the dietary potassium intake reduces the need for antihypertensive medication. Ann Intern Med 1991;115:753–759.

10a. Le QT, Elliott WJ: Dose-response relationship of blood pressure and serum cholesterol to 3-n-butyl phthalide, a component of celery oil. Clin Res 1991;39:750A.
10b. Le QT, Elliott WJ: Mechanisms of the hypotensive effect of 3-n-butyl phthalide, a component of celery oil. Clin Res 1992;40:326A.
11. Papademetriou V, Fletcher R, Khatri IM, Freis ED: Diuretic-induced hypokalemia in uncomplicated systemic hypertension: Effect of plasma potassium correction on cardiac arrhythmias. Am J Cardiol 1983;52:1017–1022.
12. Papademetriou V: Diuretics, hypokalemia and cardiac arrhythmias: A critical analysis. Am Heart J 1986;111:1217–1224.
13. Caralis PV, Materson BJ, Perez-Stable E: Potassium and diuretic-induced ventricular arrhythmias in ambulatory hypertensive patients. Min Electrolyte Metab 1984;10: 148–154.
14. Fries ED: Thiazide diuretics: How real are the concerns? [editorial]. Hosp Practice 1990;25:8–14.
15. Madias JE, Madias NE: Does diuretic-induced hypokalemia cause ventricular arrhythmias? Primary Cardiol 1987;31–41.
16. DeFronzo RA, Bonadonna RC, Ferrannini E: Pathogenesis of NIDDM. A balanced overview. Diabetic Care 1992;15:318–368.
17. Toto RD, Mitchell HC, Lee H, et al: Reversible renal insufficiency due to angiotensin converting enzyme inhibitors in hypertensive nephrosclerosis. Ann Intern Med 1991;115:513–519.
18. Lewis EJ, Hunsicker LG, Bain RP, et al: The effects of angiotensin converting enzyme inhibition in diabetic nephropathy. N Engl J Med 1993;329:1456–1462.
19. Slataper R, Vicknair R, Sadler R, et al: Comparative effects of different antihypertensive treatments on progression of diabetic renal disease. Arch Intern Med 1993;153: 973–980.
20. Bakris GL, Barnhill BW, Sadler R: Treatment of arterial hypertension in diabetic humans: Importance of therapeutic selection. Kidney Int 1992;41:912–919.
21. Brown SA, Walton CL, Crawford P, et al: Long term effects of antihypertensive regimens on renal hemodynamics and proteinuria. Kidney Int 1993;43:1210–1218.
22. Houston M: New insights and approaches to reduce end-organ damage in the treatment of hypertension: Subsets of hypertension approach. Am Heart J 1992;123:1337–1367.
23. Gibson RS, Boden WE, Theroux P, et al: Diltiazem and reinfarction in patients with non-Q wave myocardial infarction. Results of a double-blind, randomized, multicenter trial. N Engl J Med 1986;315:423–429.
24. Gibson RS: Current status of calcium channel blocking drugs after Q wave and non-Q wave myocardial infarction. Circulation 1989;80:107–119.
25. The Danish Study Group on Verapamil in Myocardial Infarction: Effect of Verapamil on mortality and major events after acute myocardial infarction. Am J Cardiol 1990;66:799–810.
26. Pepine CJ: Pharmacotherapy of myocardial infarction: Current perspectives. In Epstein M (ed): Calcium Antagonists in Clinical Medicine. Philadelphia, Hanley & Belfus, 1992, pp 165–182.
27. Klahr S, Levey AS, Beck GJ, et al: The effects of dietary protein restriction and blood pressure control on the progression of chronic renal disease. N Engl J Med 1994; 330:877–885.
28. Klahr S, Levey AS, et al: The effects of dietary protein restriction and blood pressure control on the progression of chronic renal failure. N Engl J Med 1994;330:877–885. As reported in Prevention of progression in chronic renal disease: Development of management symposium. Sponsored by the National Institute of Diabetes and Digestive and Kidney Diseases, Lister Hill Center, 1994.
29. Tolins JP, Raij L: Antihypertensive therapy and the progression of renal disease. Semin Nephrol 1991;11:538–548.
30. Wenzel UO, Helmchen U, et al: Combination treatment of enalapril with nitrendipine in rats with renovascular hypertension. Hypertension 1994;23:114–122.
31. Frohlich ED, Apstein C, Chobanian AV, et al: The heart in hypertension. N Engl J Med 1992;327:998.
32. Dahlof B, Pennert K, Hansson L: Reversal of left ventricular hypertrophy in hypertensive patients: A meta-analysis of 109 treatment studies. Am J Hypertens 1992;5:95.

33. Schulman SP, Wiess JL, Becker LC, et al: The effects of antihypertensive therapy on left ventricular mass in elderly patients. N Engl J Med 1990;322:1350–1356.
34. Frohlich ED, Horinaka S: Cardiac and aortic effects of angiotensin converting enzyme inhibitors. Hypertension 1991;18(Suppl II)II2–II7.
35. Frohlich ED: Left ventricular hypertrophy, cardiac diseases and hypertension. In Knoebel SB, Dack S (eds): An Era in Cardiovascular Medicine. New York, Elsevier, 1991, pp 85–92.
36. Neaton JD, Grimm RH, Prineas RJ, et al: Treatment of mild hypertension study: Final results. JAMA 1993;270:713–724.
37. Pfeiffer MA, Braunwald E, Moge LA, et al: Effect of captopril on mortality and morbidity in patients with left ventricular dysfunction after myocardial infarction. Results of the survival and ventricular enlargement trial. N Engl J Med 1992; 327:669.
38. Cohn JN, Johnson G, Ziesche S, et al: A comparison of enalapril with hydralazine-isosorbide dinitrate in the treatment of chronic congestive heart failure. N Engl J Med 1991;325:303.
39. The SOLVD Investigators: Effect of enalapril on mortality and the development of heart failure in asymptomatic patients with reduced left ventricular ejection fractions. N Engl J Med 1992;327:685.
40. The SOLVD Investigators: Effect of enalapril on survival in patients with reduced left ventricular ejection fractions and congestive heart failure. N Engl J Med 1991; 325:293.
40a. Gottleib SS, Dickstein K, Fleck E, et al: Hemodynamic and neurohormonal effects of the angiotensin II antagonist losartan in patients with congestive heart failure. Circulation 1993;888:1602–1609.
41. Lewis EJ, Hunsicker LG, et al: The effect of angiotensin-converting-enzyme inhibition on diabetic nephropathy. N Engl J Med 1993;329:1456–1462.
42. Bakris GL: Angiotension-converting enzyme inhibitors and progression of diabetic nephropathy [editorial]. Ann Intern Med 1993;118:643–644.
43. Mathiesen ER, Hommel E, Giese J, et al: Efficacy of captopril in postponing nephropathy in normotensive insulin dependent diabetic patients with microalbuminuria. BMJ 1991;303:81–87.
44. Ravid M, Savin H, et al: Long term stabilizing effect of angiotensin converting enzyme inhibition on plasma creatinine and on proteinuria in normotensive type II diabetic patients. Ann Intern Med 1993;118:577–581.
45. Gaber L, Walton C, Brown S, Bakris GL: Effects of different antihypertensive treatments on morphologic progression of diabetic nephropathy in uninephrectomized dogs. Kidney Int 1994;46:161–169.
46. Zeller K, Whittaker E, et al: Effect of restricting dietary protein on the progression of renal failure in patients with insulin-dependent diabetes mellitus. N Engl J Med 1991; 324:78–84.
47. Duchier J, Iannascoli F, Safar M: Antihypertensive effect of sustained release isosorbide dinitrate for isolated systolic hypertension in the elderly. Am J Cardiol 1987;60:99.
48. Giles TD, Weber M, Bartels DW, et al: Treatment of isolated systolic hypertension with labetolol in the elderly. Arch Intern Med 1990;150:974–976.
49. Barnes P: Clinical studies with calcium antagonists in asthma. Br J Clin Pharmacol 1985;20:289s.
50. Schwartzstein RS, Fanta CH: Orally administered nifedipine in chronic stable asthma. Comparison with an orally administered sympathomimetic. Am Rev Respir Dis 1986;89:959.
51. Dinh AT, Matran R, et al: Comparative effects of rilmenidine and clonidine on bronchial responses to histamine in asthmatic patients. Br J Clin Pharmacol 1988; 26:703.
52. Chodosh S, Tuck J, Pizzuto D: Prazosin in hypertensive patients with chronic bronchitis and asthma: A brief report. Am J Med 1989;86:91.
53. Lipworth BJ, McMurray JJ, Clark RA, Struthers AD: Development of late onset asthma following treatment with captopril. Eur Respir J 1989;2:586.
54. Bravo EL: Pheochromocytoma and mineralocorticoid hypertension. In Glassock RJ (ed): Current Therapy in Nephrology and hypertension, 3rd ed. St. Louis, Mosby, 1992, pp 386–391.
55. Tsapatsaris NP, Napolitana GT, Rothchild J: Osler's maneuver in an outpatient clinic setting. Arch Intern Med 1991;151:2209–2211.

CHAPTER 5

Accelerated and Malignant Hypertension

I. **Definitions**
  A. Malignant hypertension: elevated diastolic blood pressure with at least one of the following:
    1. Papilledema
    2. New central nervous system alterations:
      a. Especially abnormal mental status
      b. Differentiation from secondary hypertension due to stroke is sometimes difficult but critically important; funduscopic examination showing hemorrhages or exudates may help.
    3. New angina, myocardial infarct, or pulmonary edema
    4. Acute, progressive deterioration of renal function
  B. Accelerated hypertension: elevated diastolic blood pressure with at least one of the following:
    1. Slowly rising creatinine
    2. Progressively rising blood pressures
    3. Worsening existing end-organ damage (e.g., congestive heart failure)

II. **Cause**
  A. With preexisting hypertension
    1. Patients often 35–55 years old
  B. Secondary hypertension
    1. Birth control pills
    2. Central nervous system (e.g., cord tumors, Guillain-Barré syndrome)
    3. Acute glomerulonephritis
    4. Renovascular
    5. Withdrawal of agents, especially beta blockers and clonidine
    6. Drug interactions (*see* Appendix VIII)
      a. Monoamine oxidase inhibitors
      b. Beta blockers with clonidine or methyldopa
      c. Beta blockers with sympathomimetics
    7. Vasculitis
    8. Preeclampsia
    9. Pheochromocytoma
    10. Sympathomimetics
      a. Cocaine
      b. Amphetamines
      c. High doses of others
    11. Scleroderma

III. **Evaluation**
  A. History
    1. Medications
      a. Over-the-counter medicines
      b. Illicit drugs (cocaine, amphetamines, etc.)
      c. Psychotropics
      d. Sympathomimetic inhalers and sprays
      e. Regular medications
    2. Past history
      a. Renal
      b. Cardiac
        i. Congestive heart failure
        ii. Ischemic heart disease
      c. Central nervous system

3. Review of systems
   a. Neurologic symptoms such as
      i. Headache
      ii. Visual disturbances
      iii. Focality
      iv. Nausea or vomiting
   b. Cardiac
      i. Chest pain
      ii. Dyspnea
   c. Severe abdominal, back, neck, or chest pain may suggest aneurysm.
   d. Endocrine
      i. Paroxysms of dizziness, sweating, palpitations, headaches
      ii. Change in menstrual periods, hirsutism, amenorrhea, etc.

B. Physical examination
1. Blood pressure
   a. Right and left arms
   b. Supine and standing
   c. One leg if possible
   d. At least three readings taken several minutes apart
2. Lungs
3. Heart
4. Extremities: pulse or perfusion asymmetry
5. Neurologic
6. Fundi
7. Neck
   a. Carotid arteries
   b. Tracheal tug may be due to an aneurysm.

C. Laboratory tests
1. Electrolytes
   a. Hypokalemia is found in a large percentage of patients with malignant hypertension and may not reflect autonomous hypermineralocorticoidism.
2. Chemistry panel
3. Urinalysis
4. Electrocardiogram
5. Chest x-ray
6. Blood count
7. Blood smear (schistocytes)
8. Urine metanephrine/creatinine ratio
   a. Normal is $< 1\ \mu g/mg$.
   b. Many clinicians also do 24-hour urine measurements for metanephrine and catecholamines.

IV. **Treatment**

A. Establishment of treatment goal
1. Generally lower arterial pressure 20–25% over 4–6 hrs quickly to a mean arterial pressure of about 135 mmHg or a diastolic pressure of 100–110 mmHg.
2. Use lower pressures with aortic dissection.
3. Parenteral or rapid oral reduction of **asymptomatic "severe" high blood pressure** is almost always **not** appropriate if the patient meets no criteria for malignant hypertension.[1–5] Risk can be considerable; aggressive treatment simply based on the pressure alone is a common error.

4. Generally in primary stroke, reduction of pressure is not recommended; when reduction seems desirable, much higher pressure goals (e.g., 120 diastolic) should be considered.[6] (*See* Reactive hypertension in chapter 2.)

B. Selection of specific agents (*see also* Appendix IX)
1. Nitroprusside is usually first choice.
   a. Exceptions
      i. Aortic dissection (add beta blocker)
      ii. Pregnancy (avoid if possible)
   b. Monitor
      i. Thiocyanate levels and keep below 12 mg/dl when used more than 2 days, especially with renal impairment.
      ii. Anion gap, especially with liver impairment:
         (a) Often the first finding in cyanide toxicity.
         (b) Cyanide levels do *not* correlate with thiocyanate levels.
2. Preeclampsia (parenterally)
   a. Hydralazine
   b. Labetalol
   c. Minibolus diazoxide may be used.
   d. Calcium channel blockers under study; may interact with magnesium sulfate to cause neuromuscular blockade and/or hypertension.
   e. Nitroprusside can cause fetal cyanide toxicity and should be reserved for hypertension unresponsive to other drugs in maximal doses.
3. Sympathetic overactivity
   a. Nitroprusside
   b. Phentolamine
   c. Labetalol (not alone in pheochromocytoma, $\alpha:\beta = 1:7$ ratio)
4. Maintenance
   a. Start as soon as able.
   b. Consider calcium blockers, labetalol, and ACE inhibitors without contraindications.
   c. Many beta blockers may worsen renal blood flow.
   d. Avoid diuretics in the absence of congestive heart failure or peripheral edema early on.
5. Urgent hypertension (*see also* Appendix X)
   a. Very rapid lowering of pressure is not indicated in asymptomatic individuals.[2–5]
   b. Avoid initially large doses.
   c. Avoid normalization of pressure.
   d. Clonidine by mouth is often safest.[7]
   e. Sublingual nifedipine and ACE inhibitors have been used but may result in disproportionate hypotension and are not recommended.
6. In cocaine or amphetamine-induced hypertension, use extreme caution and short-acting drugs.

V. Drugs therapy (*see* Appendix IX)

A. Nitroprusside
1. Arteriolar and venous vasodilator
2. No change in cardiac output
3. **Starting dose:** 0.5 μg/kg/min
4. **Maintenance:** increase dose by 0.5–1 μg/kg/min every 3 minutes.

5. Hepatic or renal insufficiency: increased toxicity if used more than 2–3 days
   a. Keep thiocyanate below 10 mg/dl (100 μg/ml).
   b. Watch bicarbonate and anion gap (first abnormality in cyanide toxicity which is *not* reflected in thiocyanate levels).
   c. Antidotes
      i. Sodium nitrite
      ii. Sodium thiosulfate
      iii. Hydroxocobalamin
      iv. Hemodialysis highly effective
6. In **aortic dissection,** *must* use beta blocker first
   a. 0.5-mg test dose of propranolol over 2 minutes
   b. Then, 1 mg every 5 minutes to a maximum of 0.15 mg/kg or a heart rate of 60 bpm
   c. Maintenance: 2–6 mg every 4–6 hours

B. **Diazoxide**
1. Direct arteriolar vasodilator
2. Reflex tachycardia and increase in cardiac output
3. **Starting dose:**
   a. No prior antihypertensives: 100-mg rapid bolus
   b. Prior antihypertensives: 50–mg rapid bolus
   c. Use smaller boluses in pregnancy (*see* chapter 6).
4. Peaks in 5 minutes
5. Mainly used where constant monitoring is not possible and in pregnancy when pressure has not been responsive to other agents.

C. **Labetalol**
1. **Initial dose:**
   a. No prior drugs: 20 mg intravenously over 2 minutes
   b. Prior antihypertensives: 10 mg intravenously over 2 minutes

D. **Nonparenteral regimens** (generally not recommended) (*also see* Appendix X)
1. Nifedipine
   a. Dose: 10-mg capsule broken and liquid placed sublingually
   b. Frequency: every 30 minutes if needed
   c. Degree of pressure reduction is often unpredictable (avoid in elderly patients or those with underlying coronary or cerebrovascular disease).
2. Clonidine[7]
   a. Loading dose: 0.2 mg
   b. Further dose: 0.1 mg/hr until pressure improved or 0.7 mg total dose
3. Minoxidil and propranolol
   a. Starting dose: 10 mg of minoxidil and 40 mg of propranolol
   b. May repeat every 4 hours until goal and then go to a maintenance schedule
   c. Eventually will need loop diuretic as well
   d. Adjust beta blocker to control tachycardia.

VI. Further evaluation

In addition to the above, all patients who are suitable candidates should have a reliable evaluation for renal artery stenosis, such as magnetic resonance angiography or, preferably, intra-arterial digital subtraction renal arteriography.

REFERENCES

1. Gifford RW (chairman), et al: The fifth report of the Joint National Committee on Detection, Evaluation, and Treatment of High Blood Pressure (JNC V). Arch Intern Med 1993;153:154–183.
2. Severe symptomless hypertension [editorial]. Lancet 1989;ii:1369.
3. O'Mailia J, Sander GE, Giles TD: Nifedipine-associated myocardial ischemia or infarction in the treatment of hypertensive urgencies. Ann Intern Med 1987;107:185.
4. Zeller KR, Von Kuhnert L, Mathews C: Rapid reduction of severe asymptomatic hypertension: A prospective randomized trial. Arch Intern Med 1989;149:2186.
5. Fagan T: Acute reduction of blood pressure in asymptomatic patients with severe hypertension: An idea whose time has come—and gone [editorial]. Arch Intern Med 1989;149:2169–2170.
6. Powers WJ: Acute hypertension after stroke: The scientific basis for treatment decisions. Neurology 1993;43:461–467.
7. Anderson RJ, Hart GR, Crumpier CP, et al: Oral clonidine loading in hypertensive urgencies. JAMA 1981;246:848–850.
8. Bakris GL: Hypertension. In Stein JH (ed): Internal Medicine: Diagnosis and Therapy, 3rd ed. Norwalk, CT, Appleton, 1993; pp 171–187.

CHAPTER 6

Hypertension during Pregnancy

I. **Normal pressure and cardiac function during pregnancy**
   A. Blood pressure falls during the first half of pregnancy.
      1. Nadir mid-second trimester
      2. Falls up to 10 mmHg
      3. Normally < 75 mmHg diastolic by the end of second trimester
   B. Pressure rises during the second half of pregnancy.
      1. By the end of pregnancy, it is about equal to prepartum.
      2. Normal is defined as <85 mmHg diastolic in the third trimester.
      3. Regardless of initial pressure, a **rise of 30 mmHg systolic and/or 15 mmHg diastolic present on two occasions represents hypertension in pregnancy.**
   C. Cardiac index increases by about 50% during the first trimester and remains elevated thereafter.

II. **Incidence of hypertensive problems during pregnancy**
   A. 10% of all gestations
   B. 20% of all nulliparas
   C. 40–50% of all twinnings

III. **Classification and features**
   A. Preeclampsia-eclampsia
      1. Causes 50% of hypertension of pregnancy
      2. Onset after 20th week
      3. More in nulliparas; much less in multiparas without prior episodes
      4. Prodrome (any, all, or none of these):
         a. Headache—a sign of severe disease
         b. Severe epigastric pain—ominous
         c. Hyperreflexia
      5. Features:
         a. Hypertension
            i. May be mild.
            ii. New onset of hypertension in third trimester is grounds alone to hospitalize.
         b. Proteinuria
            i. ≥300 mg/24 hr is abnormal in pregnancy.
            ii. Early preeclampsia, especially in milder cases, may not have accompanying proteinuria.[1]
         c. Edema: It alone is not abnormal in pregnancy.
         d. Liver abnormalities and coagulation abnormalities may be present.
         e. Uric acid elevation (>4.4 mg/dl), in the absence of diuretics, is an earlier and more sensitive marker than proteinuria.[2]
         f. Eclampsia
            i. Defined as preeclampsia with seizures.
            ii. Does not necessarily correlate with the severity of the features of preeclampsia, so **all preeclamptics are at risk.**
         g. "HELLP" syndrome[3–6]
            i. Mild hypertension
            ii. Little proteinuria
            iii. Subtle hemolysis
            iv. Low platelets
            v. Abnormal liver function tests
            vi. An immediate indication of a serious problem
            vii. Immediate termination of pregnancy is very important.

viii. May become a rapidly progressive condition.
ix. Differentiation from hemolytic-uremic syndrome (HUS) and thrombotic thrombocytopenic purpura (TTP) may be difficult because of the overlap of many manifestations.
(a) HELLP almost always shows signs of resolution within 48–72 hr after termination of pregnancy.
(b) HELLP is much more common; HUS and TTP are rare.
(c) HELLP uncommonly has onset postpartum; TTP commonly begins postpartum.
(d) Fever and adenopathy are more common with HUS and TTP.
(e) Patients with HELLP often appear relatively healthy initially, with preceding laboratory abnormalities, then may deteriorate; patients with HUS and TTP usually appear critically ill from the onset of the illness.
(f) HELLP syndrome is treated with termination of pregnancy followed by supportive care; HUS/TTP is usually treated with plasma exchange.

h. Retinal arteriolar spasm (in 50% of patients)
i. Hyperreflexia
j. More common in
   i. Nulliparas
   ii. Older multiparas, especially if hypertensive
   iii. Patients living at higher altitude
   iv. Diabetes mellitus
   v. Hydatidiform mole

B. Chronic hypertension
1. Most have underlying essential hypertension.
2. Has same differential diagnosis as ordinary hypertension.
3. Has a high incidence of superimposed preeclampsia.
4. Generally accept slightly higher pressures.
5. Methyldopa is the drug of choice.
6. Patients generally do well, except
   a. Polyarteritis and collagen vascular disease have higher mortality.
   b. Significantly azotemic patients do not do well without aggressive dialytic intervention.
   c. Be sure to exclude pheochromocytoma with any suspicion.
      i. Management of pheochromocytoma patients is pharmacologic until term.[7]
   d. Hyperaldosteronemic patients may become normokalemic during pregnancy.[8]

C. Chronic hypertension with superimposed preeclampsia
1. Poorest outcome
2. High recurrence rate, even in multigravidas

D. Late or transient hypertension
1. Relatively benign condition with *no* manifestation except mild hypertension very late in pregnancy
2. A precursor of essential hypertension[3]
3. Treat as preeclampsia if any question.
4. Uric acid should be normal.

E. Late postpartum preeclampsia-eclampsia
1. Days to a week or two after delivery
2. Rare

F. Postpartum hypertension
   1. Patient is normotensive during pregnancy and becomes hypertensive weeks later, eventually normalizing within a year.

IV. **Pathophysiology in preeclampsia**
   A. Reversal of usual diurnal blood pressure variation
      1. Highest pressures at night
   B. Labile pressure
   C. Vascular hypersensitivity present, particularly to angiotensin II
   D. Decreased intravascular volume
   E. Relatively decreased cardiac output
   F. Low cardiac filling pressures
   G. Fall in renal blood flow
   H. Fall in glomerular filtration rate
   I. Impairment of escape from hyperaldosteronism that leads to sodium retention, edema, and hypertension
   J. May be caused by imbalance in endogenous vasodilators and vasoconstrictors

V. **Management of preeclampsia**
   A. Hospitalization strongly recommended
   B. If the patient normalizes in this milieu, she may occasionally be followed at home, if trustworthy.
   C. Delivery at term: **Never delay delivery at term.**
   D. Worse prognosis with any of the following[3]:
      1. Systolic pressure over 160 mmHg
      2. Diastolic pressure over 110 mmHg
      3. Protein excretion >2 gm/24 hr or spot urine protein >100 mg/dl
      4. Increasing serum creatinine
      5. Evidence of hemolysis including schistocytes, high lactate dehydrogenase (LDH)
      6. Epigastric or right upper abdominal pain
      7. Severe headache or other central nervous system signs
      8. Congestive heart failure
      9. Retinal hemorrhages, exudates, or papilledema; the presence of these signs without any other adverse prognostic finding may suggest underlying preexistent chronic hypertension.[3]
      10. Intrauterine growth retardation
   E. In patients who have not yet reached 34 weeks, an attempt may be made to stabilize
      1. If attempts to keep diastolic blood pressure below 105 mmHg (100 in teenagers) fail after 24–48 hours, delivery by cesarian section is mandatory anyway.
      2. *Never* delay delivery if these appear:
         a. Worsening headache
         b. Worsening or severe epigastric pain
         c. Worsening or persistent hyperreflexia
         d. Failure to control blood pressure, as above
         e. Clotting abnormality, especially thrombocytopenia
         f. Liver function abnormalities
   F. Approach to treatment
      1. To what level?
         a. Controversial
         b. Approximately 90–105 mmHg diastolic
         c. Too low may also be harmful.

TABLE 9. Use of Magnesium Sulfate in the Treatment of Preeclampsia

5 gm intravenous piggyback over 10 min	Decrease for hyporeflexia pending levels.
Then 1 gm/hr	Continue administration for 24 hr postpartum.
Keep levels between 6 and 9 mg/dl.	Keep an ampule of calcium gluconate at bedside for emergency treatment of hypermagnesemia.
Increase dose for hyperreflexia.	

2. Bedrest: important to include some ambulation to avoid deep vein thrombosis[9]
3. Treatment of choice in patients past 34–36 weeks is *always* immediate delivery.
4. If patient has **altered mentation, neurologic findings, altered liver function tests, or low platelets, deliver at any stage** since baby has a better chance outside a toxemic uterus.
5. First drug of choice in the absence of severe tachycardia is hydralazine, 5 mg intravenously and then 5–10 mg intravenously every 20–30 minutes.
6. Many physicians now use parenteral labetalol next: 20 mg intravenous bolus every 10 min to maximum of 300 mg. Follow bolus control with infusion 1–2 mg/min (20–40 cc/hr of 800 mg/250 cc concentration).
7. Miniboluses of diazoxide 30 mg also may be used.
8. Magnesium sulfate is used in most cases as an adjunct and to prevent seizures; it should be continued 24 hours postpartum (Table 9). It may interact with calcium channel blockers to cause hypotension or neuromuscular blockade.
9. Although safe by some studies, beta blockers (other than labetalol) have not been as well studied and may impair stress tolerance of the fetus.
10. Avoid all other medications; many are of unknown toxicity. The following drugs are **contraindicated:**
    a. Nitroprusside (except when the above fail)
    b. ACE inhibitors[10,11]
    c. Ganglionic blockers
11. Although volume expansion was once advocated, it is no longer recommended because[12–15]
    a. Myocardial performance may be compromised.
    b. Volume expansion with sodium may increase vascular reactivity.
    c. The administration of nonprotein fluid decreases oncotic pressure which may lead to pulmonary edema and cerebral edema.
12. Volume expansion with colloid may be used when it seems mandatory, but only with monitoring of central pressures.
13. Do liver ultrasound on any patient with persistent abdominal pain to rule out subcapsular hemorrhage (which may be fatal if untreated).
14. Diuretics are avoided except as a last resort or with frank congestive heart failure; if fluid retention *due to medications* occurs, diuretics may be used *with caution.*
15. Chronic hypertension in the absence of preeclampsia:
    a. 85% of patients do fine.
    b. More complications occur in patients over 30.
    c. Methyldopa is still the drug of choice in pregnancy for treatment of chronic hypertension.
    d. Diuretics are generally avoided acutely but can be continued chronically if the patient was salt-sensitive prior to pregnancy.
    e. Use of beta blockers and labetalol may be associated with fetal growth retardation if used in early pregnancy.[16]

VI. **Prevention**

Only low-dose aspirin has been shown (in small studies) to prevent preeclampsia. These are preliminary studies and this treatment should probably be reserved for patients with prior preeclampsia and high risk of recurrence (e.g., a patient with chronic essential hypertension over age 40 with a history of preeclampsia).[17-20]

VII. **Follow up**

A. Evaluations at 3 months postpartum (in **all** patients):
   1. Blood pressure
   2. 24-hour urine protein
   3. Urine sediment

B. All manifestations should have resolved by then. Abnormal findings indicate an underlying disease such as chronic glomerulonephritis. These patients should be evaluated by a nephrologist.[2]

REFERENCES

1. Brown MA, Whitworth JA: The kidney in hypertensive pregnancies—Victim and villain. Am J Kidney Dis 1992;20:427–442.
2. Chua S, Redmond CWG: Prognosis for pre-eclampsia complicated by 5 g or more of proteinuria in 24 hours. Eur J Obstet Gynecol Reprod Biol 1992;43:9–12.
3. Pritchard JA, Weisman R, Ratnoff OD, Vosburgh GJ: Intravascular hemolysis, thrombocytopenia and other hematologic abnormalities associated with severe toxemia of pregnancy. N Engl J Med 1954;250:89–98.
4. Weinstein L: Syndrome of hemolysis, elevated liver enzymes, and low platelet count: A severe consequence of hypertension in pregnancy. Am J Obstet Gynecol 1982;142:159–167.
5. Killam AP, Dillard SH, Patton RC, Pederson PR: Pregnancy-induced hypertension complicated by acute liver disease and disseminated intravascular coagulation: Five case reports. Am J Obstet Gynecol 1975;123:823–828.
6. Miller JM, Pastorek JG: Thrombotic thrombocytopenic purpura and hemolytic uremic syndrome in pregnancy. Clin Obstet Gynecol 1991;34:64–71.
7. Lindheimer MD: Hypertension in pregnancy. Hypertension 1993;22:127–137.
8. August P, Sealey JE: The renin-angiotensin system in normal and hypertensive pregnancy, and ovarian function. In Laragh JH, Brenner BM (eds): Hypertension: Pathophysiology, Diagnosis and Management. New York, Raven Press, 1990, pp 1761–1768.
9. Brown MA: Nonpharmacological management of pregnancy induced hypertension. J Hyperten 1990;8:295–301.
10. Are ACE inhibitors safe in pregnancy [editorial]? Lancet 1989;ii:482–483.
11. Hennessey A, Horvath JS: Newer antihypertensive agents in pregnancy. Med J Aust 1992;156:304–305.
12. Sibai BM, et al: Pulmonary edema in severe preeclampsia-eclampsia: Analysis of thirty-seven consecutive cases. Am J Obstet Gynecol 1984;156:1174–1179.
13. Benedetti TJ, Kates R, Williams V: Hemodynamic observations in severe preeclampsia complicated by pulmonary edema. Am J Obstet Gynecol 1985;152:330–334.
14. Benedetti TJ, Quilligan EJ: Cerebral edema in severe pregnancy-induced hypertension. Am J Obstet Gynecol 1980;137:860–862.
15. Pritchard JA, Cunningham FG, Pritchard SA: The Parkland Memorial Hospital Protocol for treatment of eclampsia: Evaluation of 245 cases. Am J Obstet Gynecol 1984;148:951–963.
16. Sturgis SN, Lindheimer MD, Davison JM: Treatment of hypertension during pregnancy: Drugs to be avoided and drugs to be used. In Andreucci VE, Fine LG (eds): International Yearbook of Nephrology. New York, Springer-Verlag, 1991, pp 163–196.
17. Beaufuls M, Uzan S, Donsimoni, Colau. Prevention of preeclampsia by early antiplatelet therapy. Lancet 1985;i:840–842.
18. Wallenberg HCS, Dekker GA, Makovitz JW, Rotmans P: Low dose aspirin prevents pregnancy-induced hypertension and preeclampsia in angiotensin-sensitive primigravidae. Lancet 1986; i:1–3.
19. Benigni A, Gregorini G, Frusca T, et al: Effect of low-dose aspirin on fetal and maternal generation of thromboxane by platelets in women at risk for pregnancy induced hypertension. N Engl J Med 1989;321:357–362.
20. Schiff E, Peleg E, Goldenberg M, et al: The use of aspirin to prevent pregnancy-induced hypertension and lower the ratio of thromboxane A_2 to prostacyclin in relatively high-risk pregnancies. N Engl J Med 1986;321:351–356.

APPENDIX I

Approach to the Patient with Suspected Cushing's Syndrome

APPENDIX I

Approach to the Patient with Suspected Cushing's Syndrome

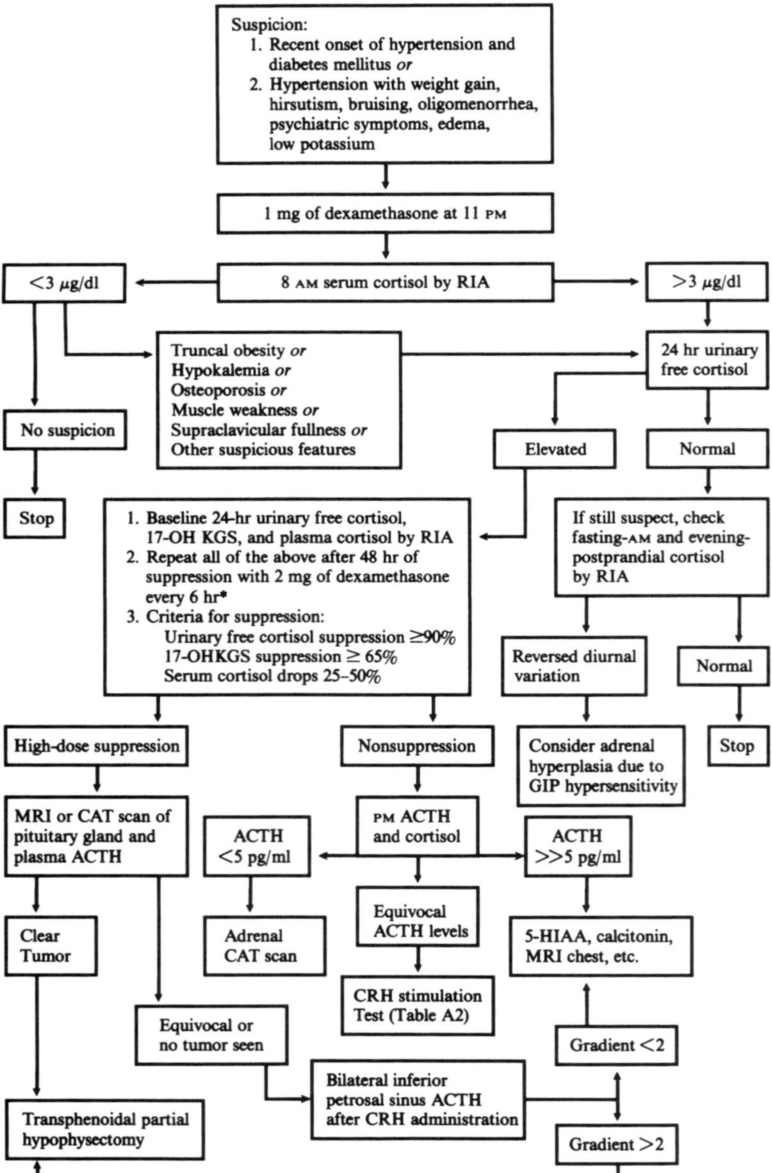

* A high-dose overnight test uses a single 8-mg dose of dexamethasone followed by a plasma cortisol the following morning; this test is an alternative (though not as established).

TABLE A1. False Results in the Overnight Dexamethasone Suppression Test and Urinary Free Cortisol Test

Overnight Dexamethasone Suppression Test		Urinary Free Cortisol Test
False-positives	**False-negatives**	**False-positives**
Common	Ketoconazole	Uncommon
Acute psychiatric stress		Diuretics
Depression		High sodium diet
Uncommon		
Diphenylhydantoin (phenytoin)		
Alcohol		
Rifampin		
Birth control pills		

The patient who is suspected of having Cushing's syndrome will have some or all of the characteristics listed at the top of the chart. A simple screening test is the overnight dexamethasone suppression test. False-positives do occur with varying frequency (Table A1). To improve reliability, use only **radioimmunoassay measurements of cortisol**. With high suspicion, however, this should not be relied on to rule out the diagnosis absolutely. In this case, a 24-hour urinary free cortisol is usually diagnostic.

If the patient has a normal urinary cortisol in the face of convincing clinical findings suggestive of Cushing's syndrome, a check of the plasma cortisol for reversal of the normal diurnal variation may be useful. If the afternoon value is higher than the fasting value, this is suggestive of the syndrome of gastric inhibitory peptide (GIP) hypersensitivity.[1,2] If urinary free cortisol is elevated, 24-hour urinary free cortisol, 17-hydroxy corticosteroids (17-OHKGS = 17-hydroxy-ketogenic steroids) and plasma cortisol are measured before and after high-dose dexamethasone suppression (given as 2 mg every 6 hours). If urinary free cortisol is suppressed $\geq 90\%$ along with suppression of 17-hydroxy steroids $\geq 65\%$, pituitary Cushing's syndrome is strongly suspected. An overnight high-dose dexamethasone suppression test has recently been described and seems reliable. The difficulties with this test are the relatively small number of patients studied and the fact that it has been validated only in hospitalized patients.[3–5] Nonsuppression leads to measurement of adrenocorticotrophic hormone (ACTH) and search for ectopic secretion of the ACTH. These tests include hydroxyindoleacetic acid (5-HIAA) for carcinoid tumors and magnetic resonance imaging (MRI) of the chest and/or other appropriate locations. Computed tomography (CT) scanning

TABLE A2. The CRH Stimulation Test[4]

Protocol

1. Obtain baseline ACTH and cortisol levels.
2. Administer 1 μg/kg or 100 μg of CRH at about 8:00 AM.
3. Obtain blood samples for ACTH and cortisol at 15-minute intervals for at least 2 hours.
4. Test valid only in untreated state.

Interpretation

1. Normal: Flat or slightly rising curve; normal baseline ACTH.
2. Pituitary: Sharp rise in ACTH (even to fivefold or more) with concomitant rise in cortisol; usually elevated baseline ACTH.
3. Adrenal: Relatively flat curve; suppressed baseline ACTH.
4. Ectopic ACTH: Relatively flat curve; higher baseline ACTH.

and MRI are probably equivalent for pituitary imaging in the case of high-dose suppression. Failure to see a clear tumor under this circumstance justifies sampling of bilateral inferior petrosal sinus ACTH levels after administration of corticotropin-releasing factor (CRF). Lack of a difference between the two sides leads to further search for the unusual ectopic ACTH source which is suppressible.

REFERENCES

1. Reznick YR, Veronigue A, Chayvialle JA, et al: Food dependent Cushing's syndrome mediated by aberrant adrenal sensitivity to gastric inhibitory polypeptide. N Engl J Med 1992;327:981–986.
2. Lacroix A, Bolte E, Tremblay J, et al: Gastric inhibitory polypeptide-dependent cortisol hypersecretion—A new cause of Cushing's syndrome. N Engl J Med 1992;327:974–980.
3. Tyrell JB, Findling JW, et al: An overnight high-dose dexamethasone suppression test in the aetiological diagnosis of Cushing's syndrome. Acta Endocrinol (Copenhagen) 1984;109:158–162.
4. Bruno OD, Rossi MA, et al: Nocturnal high-dose dexamethasone suppression test in the aetiological diagnosis of Cushing's syndrome. Acta Endocrinol (Copenhagen) 1985;109:158–162.
5. Kaye TB, Crapo L: The Cushing syndrome: An update on diagnostic tests. Ann Intern Med 1990;112:434–444.
6. Findling JW, Mazzaferri EL: Cushing syndrome—An etiologic workup. Hosp Pract 1992;27:107–122.
7. Orth DN: Cushing's syndrome. N Engl J Med 1995;332:791–803.

APPENDIX II

Approach to the Patient with Suspected Hyperaldosteronism

APPENDIX II

Approach to the Patient with Suspected Hyperaldosteronism

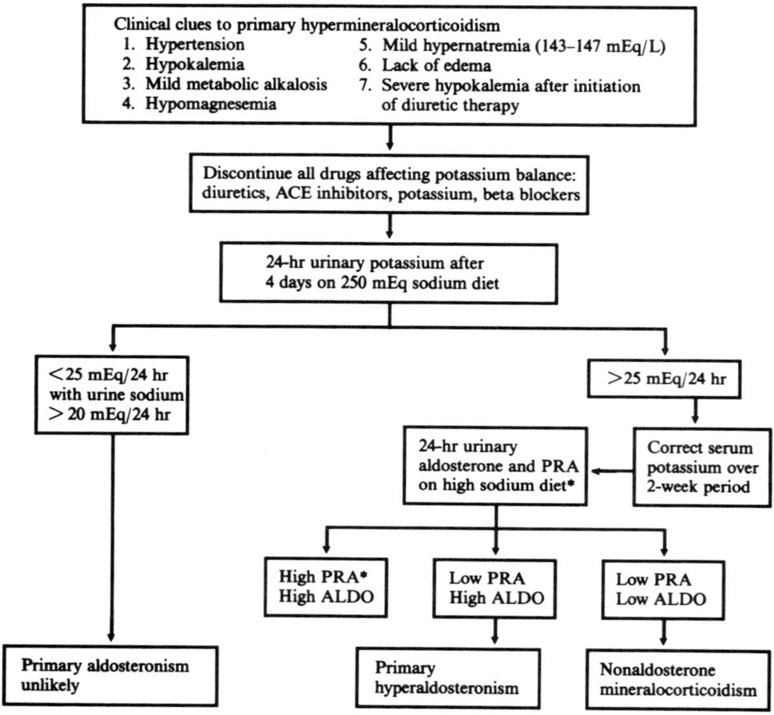

FIGURE A2. Initial evaluation of the patient with suspected hypermineralocorticoidism. The evaluation of the patient with suspected hyperaldosteronism starts with clinical suspicion. This may include any or all of the factors listed. Mild hypokalemia while on diuretics by itself is not grounds for further evaluation. On the other hand, some patients with various forms of hypermineralocorticoidism may be normokalemic, especially on a sodium-restricted diet. The majority of patients with *correctable* disease are believed to be hypokalemic, however.

Evaluation starts with a 24-hour urinary sodium and potassium determination. If urinary potassium is low (<25–30 mEq/24 hr) in the presence of adequate salt intake (>200 mEq/day off of diuretics), this excludes hypermineralocorticoidism. If elevated, the next step is to evaluate the renin-aldosterone axis after potassium repletion (potassium is a major regulator of aldosterone secretion). In many cases of primary hyperaldosteronism, aldosterone (ALDO) will be unsuppressed and renin suppressed; however, in some patients with proven primary hyperaldosteronism, plasma renin activity (PRA) may not suppress (**see* Fig. A3). Patients with inappropriate kaliuresis while on a high-salt diet who have suppressed aldosterone should be investigated for alternative mineralocorticoids if they do not have another explanation (such as estrogen administration, renovascular disease, malignant hypertension, or salt-wasting nephropathy—*see* Fig. A4, Table A6). Note that aldosterone secretion is suppressed by hypokalemia and that this will overcome the effects of distal sodium delivery on potassium excretion in normal people.[2,3] Patients with high plasma renin activity and high aldosterone may have renal artery stenosis or, rarely, a renin-secreting tumor of the kidney (perihemangiocytoma) or ectopic secretion of renin from another tumor (e.g., oat cell carcinoma of the lung.)

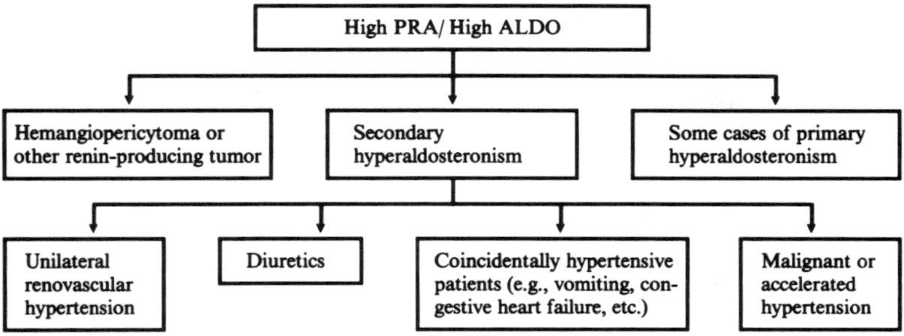

FIGURE A3. Differential diagnosis of hypokalemic hypertensive patients with high plasma renin activity and high aldosterone levels.

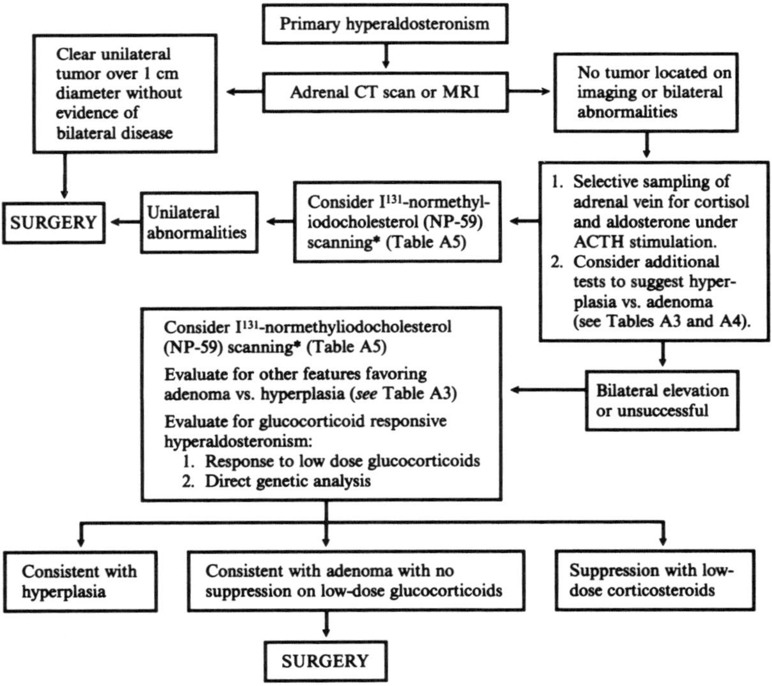

FIGURE A4. **Approach to the patient with confirmed hyperaldosteronism.** The evaluation of a patient with confirmed hyperaldosteronism requires further testing to determine if the cause is primary adrenal hyperplasia, a solitary adenoma, or glucocorticoid-suppressible hyperaldosteronism (GSHA). Since GSHA is uncommon, even small adrenal tumors must be excluded first (with adrenal vein aldosterone if necessary). When adrenal venous sampling is done, high ACTH-stimulated cortisol relative to mixed blood, in each adrenal vein specimen, assures the physician that the specimen was indeed obtained from the adrenal vein. Because bilateral abnormalities on MRI or CT may not represent functional adrenal hyperplasia, the diagnosis in such circumstances should be confirmed with additional tests such as those in Table A3 and/or an I^{131}-iodocholesterol scan.*

*These tests are not widely available.

TABLE A3. Tests in the Differentiation of Adrenal Hyperplasia vs Solitary Adrenal Adenoma

Test	Bilateral	Unilateral
Plasma aldosterone change with upright posture (Table A4)	Increased	Decreased
Ratio of 18-hydroxycorticosterone to cortisol after normal saline infusion over 2 hr	<3	>3
Urinary hydroxycortisol*	Low	High
Urinary aldosterone response to spironolactone	Increased	Decreased

* These tests not widely available.

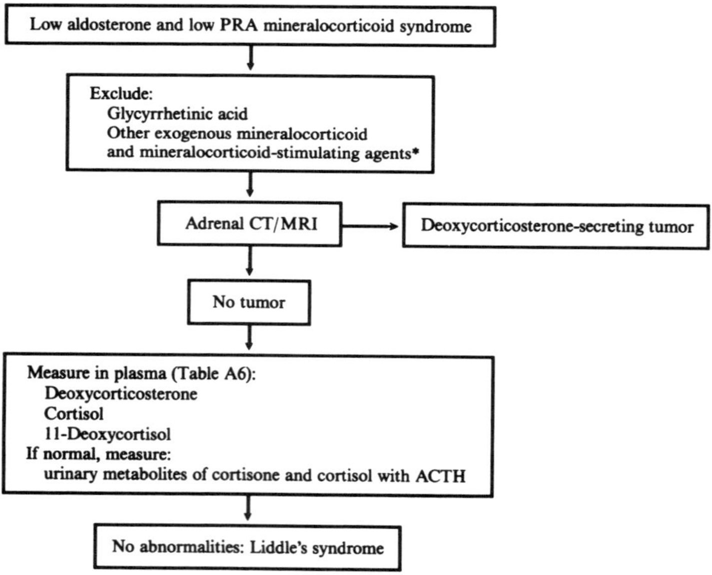

FIGURE A5. Evaluation of the patient with suspected hyperaldosteronism and low renin and aldosterone. * Mineralocorticoid-stimulating agents include carbenoxolone, fluorinated steroids, licorice, and licorice-flavored tobacco, laxatives, and beverages.

TABLE A4. Protocol for Determination of Postural Variation in Plasma Aldosterone

Protocol for Postural Aldosterone Studies	Interpretation of Results
1. Discontinue spironolactone* and ACE inhibitors. 2. Place patient on a 150 mEq day (3.5 g Na) diet for 5 days. 3. Place patient in lying position overnight. 4. At 7 AM without arising, place indwelling catheter. 5. Draw 8 AM plasma aldosterone, 18-hydroxy-corticosterone, potassium, cortisol and PRA. 6. Ambulate and collect upright specimens at noon.	1. Normal patients have a 2- to 4-fold rise in aldosterone. 2. Patients with hyperplasia have at least a 33% rise in aldosterone. 3. Patients with unilateral adenomas have little or no change. 4. The test is invalid if cortisol fails to decrease with the noon measurement.

* Spironolactone should be discontinued for 6 weeks prior to study.

TABLE A5. I^{131}-Methylnoriodocholesterol (NP59) Scanning

1. Give dexamethasone 1 mg by mouth four times a day starting one week prior to isotope injection; continue for a total of ten days (to suppress normal adrenal tissue).
2. Starting 2 days prior to isotope injection, give 1 drop SSKI by mouth three times a day; continue for 2 weeks (to protect thyroid).
3. Inject 5mCi of ^{131}I-Iodomethyl-19-norcholesterol (NP59) 1 week after initiation of dexamethasone and 3 days after initiation of SSKI.
4. Intercurrent ^{99m}Tc-DTPA or glucoheptonate scans may be used for anatomic reference.
5. Some authors recommend a routine radiological bowel preparation.
6. Interpretation of results:
   a. Bilateral uptake usually seen in hyperplasia.
   b. Unilateral hot area usually seen with adenoma.
   c. Carcinoma often cold bilaterally.

TABLE A6. Tests in the Differential Diagnosis of Nonaldosterone Mineralocorticoidism

Entity	Cortisol	Deoxycorticosterone	11-Deoxycortisol	Cortisol Metabolites	Cortisone Metabolites
Licorice	N	N	N	H	L
Apparent mineralocorticoid excess syndrome	N	N	N	H	L
11-beta hydroxylase deficiency	L	H	H	L	—
17-hydroxylase deficiency	L	H	L	L	—
Cortisol resistance	H	H	H	H	H

TABLE A7. Summary of Test Results in Apparent Hypermineralocorticoid States

	[K]	PRA	ALDO	ACTH	17-KS	RVR	DOC
Primary hyperaldosteronism	L/N	L	H	N	N	N	L
Glucocorticoid-responsive hyperaldosteronism	N/L	L	H	H/N	N	N	L
Cushing's syndrome	N/L	N/H	N/H	N/H	N/H	N	N/H
Liddle's syndrome	L	L	L	N	N	N	N
11-OH deficiency	N/L	L	L	N/H	H	—	H
17-OH deficiency	L	L	L	N/H	L	—	H
DOC tumor	L	L	L	L/N	N	—	H
Licorice	L	L	L	N	N	N	N
Hemangiopericytoma and ectopic renin	L	H	H	N	N	N/H	H
Renovascular hypertension	N/L	N/H	N/H	N	N	N/H	N

[K] = serum potassium; PRA = plasma renin activity; ALDO = aldosterone; ACTH = adrenocorticotrophic hormone; 17-KS = 17-ketosteroids; RVR = renal vein renin; DOC = deoxycorticosterone; N = normal; H = high; and L = low.

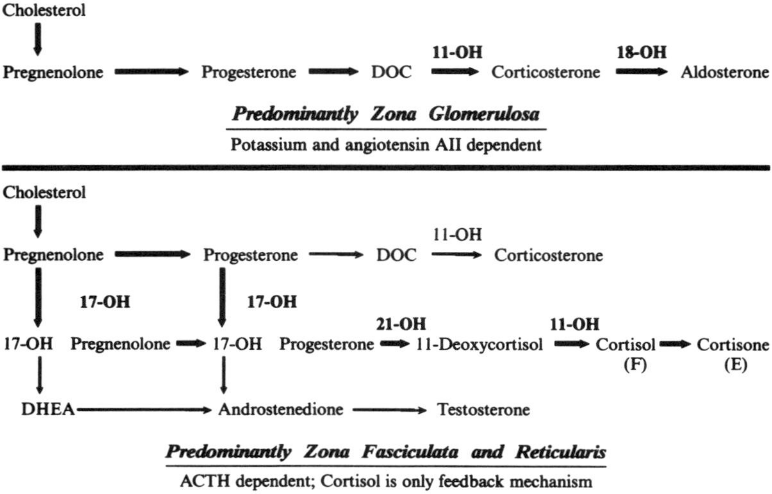

FIGURE A6. Metabolic pathways and defects in hypermineralocorticoid states. Heavy arrows indicate normal major pathways; light arrows indicate minor pathways which may become important in certain disease states.

1. ACTH stimulates the adrenal cortex, which results in increased production of cortisol which, in turn, feeds back to suppress secretion of ACTH.
2. Angiotensin II stimulates the secretion of aldosterone.
3. Failure of cortisol production for any reason leads to increased ACTH release and therefore increased synthesis of steroids up to the point in the metabolic pathways where the enzyme involved is deficient or inhibited.
4. Because 21-hydroxylase (21-OH) deficiency blocks the pathway to all mineralocorticoids, patients with this disorder have a tendency toward hyperkalemia and are normotensive or even salt-wasting. Androgens also accumulate.
5. In 11-hydroxylase (11-OH) deficiency, deoxycorticosterone (DOC), a potent mineralocorticoid, and 11-deoxycortisol accumulate as do the androgens.
6. In 17-hydroxylase (17-OH) deficiency, not only does deoxycorticosterone accumulate, but the pathway to sex steroids is blocked as is that to cortisol.
7. Normally, aldosterone is produced only in the zona glomerulosa and not in the zona fasciculata, where ACTH acts preferentially; in glucocorticoid-responsive hyperaldosteronism, aldosterone synthase, a specific 18-hydroxylase usually limited to the zona glomerulosa, is present in the zona fasciculata; this causes ordinary ACTH secretion to stimulate aldosterone synthesis. The disorder is treated with ACTH suppression via exogenous glucocorticoid. 18-OH = 18-hydroxylase; DHEA = dihydroxyepiandrosterone.

REFERENCES

1. Biglieri EG: Spectrum of mineralocorticoid hypertension. Hypertension 1991;17:251–261.
2. Rose BD: Clinical Physiology of Acid-Base and Electrolyte Disorders, 3rd ed. New York, McGraw-Hill, 1993, pp 722–730.
3. Bravo EL, Tarazi RC, Dustan H, et al: The changing clinical spectrum of primary hyperaldosteronism. Am J Med 1983;74:641–651.
4. Bakris GL, Mazzaferri EL: Severe hypertension in a young patient. Hosp Pract 1993; 28:57–64.
5. Slataper RM, Bakris GL: Secondary hypertension. In Taylor R (ed): Difficult Diagnosis II. Philadelphia, W.B. Saunders, 1992, pp 403–411.
6. Young WF, Hogan MJ, Klee GG, et al: Primary aldosteronism: Diagnosis and treatment. Mayo Clin Proc 1990;65:96–110.

APPENDIX III

Workup and Management of Pheochromocytoma

APPENDIX III

Workup and Management of Pheochromocytoma

I. **Approach to diagnosis of a pheochromocytoma (Fig. A7)**

A. In patients in whom the diagnosis of pheochromocytoma is suspected, **24-hour urinary normetanephrine assay** is the most reliable single test,[1] with total metanephrine also being a consistently good test.[2] Vanillylmandelic acid (VMA) and urinary catecholamines are less sensitive and have both lower sensitivity and low specificity; however, measurement of *free* (not total) urinary catecholamines and VMA by *fluorometric assay after HPLC* (high-pressure liquid chromotography) separation have much greater reliability than older, but still commonly employed methods.[3] In this regard, it is important to know which assays are being used with HPLC methods. Table A8 lists tests with high reliability.

TABLE A8. Interpretation of 24-Hour Urinary Results in Patients with Suspected Pheochromocytoma

Test	Normal Values	Usual in Pheochromocytoma	Interference
Normetanephrine (Fluorometric assay)	≤0.720 mg/24 hr	>2 mg/24 hr (Values <720 mg/24 hr are rare.)	Monoamine oxidase inhibitors Beta blockers Exogenous catecholamines Tetracyclines Acetaminophen
Total metanephrines	≤1.3 mg/24 hr	>2 mg/24 hr	Same as normetanephrine
Vanillylmandelic acid (best after HPLC)	≤7 mg/24 hr	>14 mg/24 hr	Carbidopa Methyldopa Clofibrate Disulfiram Monoamine oxidase inhibitors Carbidopa-levodopa Reserpine Nitroglycerin Exogenous catecholamines
Urinary *free* epinephrine + norepinephrine (not conjugated) Catecholamines (best after HPLC)	<150 μg/24 hr	≥240 μg/24 hr	Methyldopa Ganglionic blockers Radiographic dye Reserpine Catecholamines Acetaminophen Alcohol L-DOPA Methenamine Nicotine Nitroglycerin Erythromycin Tetracyclines Theophylline B vitamins in large doses Beta blockers Bananas

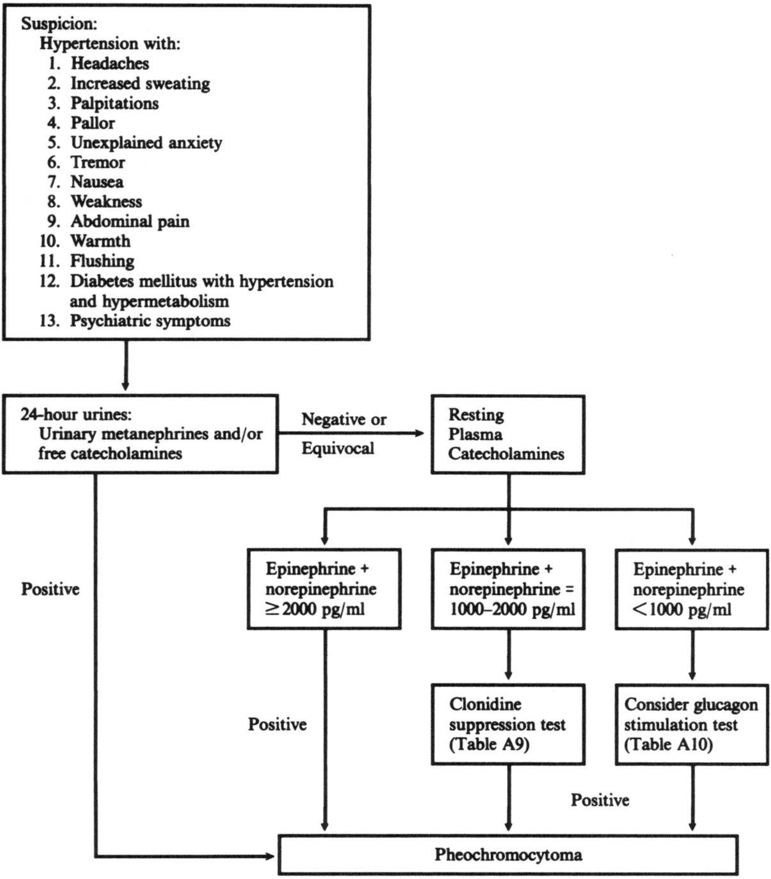

FIGURE A7. Approach to diagnosis of pheochromocytoma.

TABLE A9. Clonidine Suppression Test[4,5,6]

Procedure[4,5]

1. Discontinue antihypertensives 12 hr prior to test.
2. Be sure patient is volume repleted.
3. Place heparin lock for blood drawing 30 min before drawing blood.
4. 30 min after heparin lock is inserted, draw baseline plasma catecholamines; put blood on ice.
5. Administer 0.3 mg of clonidine by mouth.
6. Redraw three more plasma catecholamine specimens at 1-hr intervals over the next 3 hr.

Interpretation

1. Normal suppression by 50% to <500 pg/ml.
2. Results are invalid without elevated resting level.[6]
3. Volume repletion prior to test is mandatory or profound hypotension may result.

TABLE A10. The Glucagon Stimulation Test*

Procedure[1,5,7,8]
1. Pretreat patient with alpha blocker or calcium channel blocker.
2. Place heparin lock for blood drawing 30 min prior to test.
3. Draw baseline plasma catecholamines.
4. Give 1 mg of intravenous glucagon.

Interpretation
1. Pheochromocytoma patients have a 3-fold or greater increase in catecholamines *or* an absolute value > 2000 μg/ml.

* For patients suspected of having a pheochromocytoma but with catecholamines below 1000 pg/mL.

B. During **paroxysms**, patients may be asked to empty their bladder for a double-voided spot **urinary metanephrine/creatinine ratio.**
   1. Test urine metanephrine/creatinine ratio while hypertensive.
   2. Values over 1 μg/mg (metanephrine/creatinine) are abnormal.
   3. Particularly useful as a double-voided specimen following a rise in pressure.
   4. Should be confirmed with fractionated urinary 24-hour tests.

C. **Plasma catecholamines** are useful in confirming the diagnosis, especially in equivocal cases:
   1. Procedure: patient is resting, supine; heparin lock in place 1 hour prior to test.
   2. Diagnostic:
      a. Norepinephrine > 2000 pg/ml (12 nmol/L)
      b. Epinephrine > 200 pg/ml (1.1 nmol/L)
   3. Nondiagnostic elevations can be caused by
      a. Anxiety
      b. Smoking
      c. Exercise
      d. Pheochromocytoma
   4. Potentially useful in borderline cases, especially with clonidine suppression, which does not suppress the result in pheochromocytoma.

II. **Localization of pheochromocytomas (Fig. A8)**

A. Because 5% of pheochromocytomas occur in the setting of multiple endocrine neoplasia syndrome type II (MEN-II), beware of the possibility of medullary carcinoma of the thyroid as well as hyperparathyroidism.
B. Computed tomography (CT) is positive in detecting 90% of cases.
C. Because bladder tumors are a common site of extra-adrenal tumors, intravenous pyelography with views of the bladder may be valuable if the CT scanning is not diagnostic.
D. ^{131}I-metaiodobenzylguanidine (MIBG) scans can pick up most of the rest, but are not widely available (Table A11).
E. Scanning of the mediastinum and rarely elsewhere may be needed.
F. Occasionally, adrenal venographic sampling is still necessary.

III. **Preoperative management of pheochromocytoma**

A. First, a long-acting alpha blocker (phenoxybenzamine) is used to maximally inhibit postsynaptic alpha receptors (as evidenced by ≥ 20 mmHg drop in blood pressure after standing).

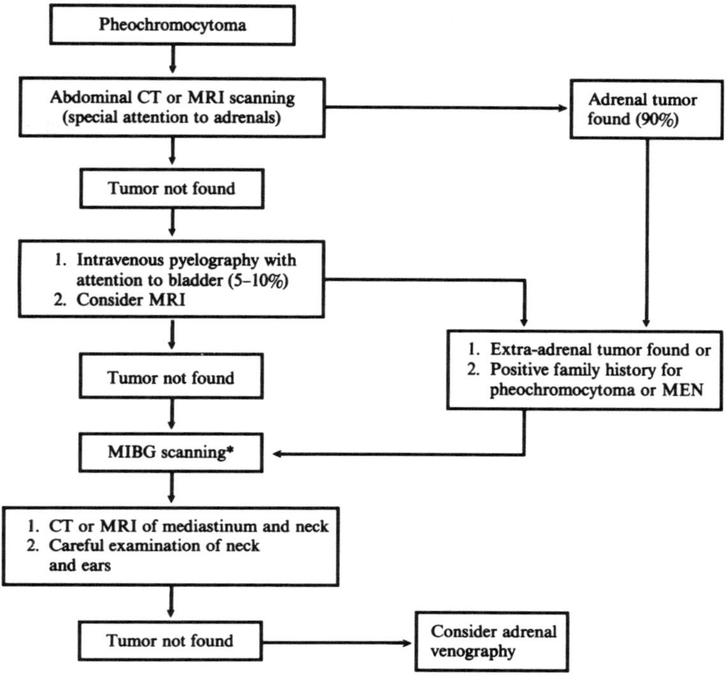

FIGURE A8. Approach to localization of pheochromocytoma. * Available at very few centers.

B. Calcium blockers can then be added; beta blockade may occasionally be needed in patients with high epinephrine-like activity, *but only after maximal alpha blockade.*

C. Volume expansion preoperatively is *critical.*
   1. These patients have the greatest need for volume expansion compared to those with other causes of secondary hypertension.
   2. Give at least 2–5 L of normal saline.
   3. Administer under hemodynamic monitoring, if necessary.

IV. Beware of factitious exogenous catecholamine administration in strange cases, especially among health professionals.

TABLE A11. ^{131}-I-meta-iodobenzylguanidine (MIBG) Scanning for Localization of Pheochromocytoma

1. Screen for factors which may interfere with test (reserpine; phenothiazines; labetalol; cocaine; tricyclic antidepressants; pseudoephedrine, phenylpropanolamine, other sympathomimetic amines; amphetamines; ?chocolate; ?vanilla; ?clonidine; ?certain cheeses) and substitute for interfering drugs at least 24 hr in advance.
2. Give 100 mg of iodide as Lugol's solution or SSKI at time of isotope administration.
3. Administer 7–14 uCi/Kg of ^{131}I MIBG.
4. Do scan 24 hr after ^{131}I MIBG; include skull through pelvis.

REFERENCES

1. DeQuattro V, Meyers M, Campese VM: Pheochromocytoma: Diagnosis and therapy. In Degroot LJ, Besser GM, Cahill GF, et al (eds): Endocrinology. Philadelphia, W.B. Saunders, 1989, pp 1780–1797.
2. Manu P, Runge LA: Biochemical screening for pheochromocytoma: Superiority of urinary metanephrines measurements. Am J Epidemiol 1984;120:788–790.
3. Stein PP, Black HR: A simplified diagnostic approach to pheochromocytoma: A review of the literature and report of one institution's experience. Medicine 1990;70:46–66.
4. Bravo EL, Terazi RC, Fouad F, et al: Clonidine suppression test. A useful aid in the diagnosis of pheochromocytoma. N Engl J Med 1981;305:623–626.
5. Grossman E, Goldstein DS, Hoffman A, Keiser HR: Glucagon and clonidine testing in the diagnosis of pheochromocytoma. Hypertension 1991;17:733–741.
6. Elliot WJ, Murphy MB: Reduced specificity of the clonidine suppression test in patients with normal plasma catecholamine levels. Am J Med 1988;84:419–424.
7. Sheps SG, Jiang N, Klee GG, et al: Recent developments in the diagnosis and treatment of pheochromocytoma. Mayo Clin Proc 1990;65:88–95.
8. Bravo EM: Pheochromocytoma: New concepts and future trends. Kidney Int 1991;40:544–556.
9. Setaro JF, Black HR: Current concepts: Refractory hypertension. N Engl J Med 1992;327:543–547.

APPENDIX IV

Approach to the Patient with Suspected Renovascular Hypertension

APPENDIX IV

Approach to the Patient with Suspected Renovascular Hypertension

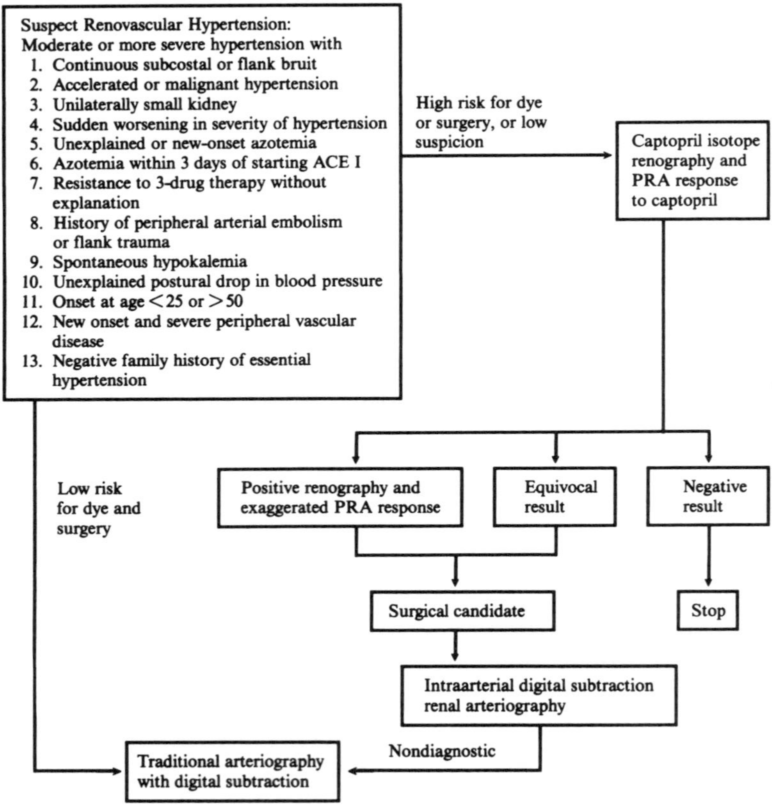

FIGURE A9. Evaluation of the patient with suspected renovascular hypertension. Protocols for isotopic renography and plasma renin activity (PRA) determinations are shown in Tables A12 and A13.

TABLE A12. Protocol for Captopril Isotopic Renography with Simultaneous Assay of Plasma Renin Activity

1. Stop ACE inhibitors 24 hr prior to test; stop diuretics 1 wk prior to test if possible; check urine sodium to confirm patient is sodium replete.
2. Give 24 oz of water 1 hr prior to test.
3. Check blood pressure and PRA.
4. Give 50 mg of crushed oral captopril by mouth.*
5. One hr later, draw repeat sitting PRA and do DTPA renography.

* Because of severe postural hypotension after captopril administration in some patients, it may become necessary to administer intravenous saline.

DTPA = ^{99m}Tc-diethylenetriaminepentaacetate.

TABLE A13. Interpretion of Plasma Renin Activity Accompanying Captopril Isotropic Renography

Criteria for positive PRA results (sodium-replete)
1. Stimulated PRA of ≥ 12 μg/L/hr (ng/cc/hr **and**
2. Increase of PRA by 10 μg/L/hr (ng/cc/hr) **and**
3. Increase in PRA by 150% or 400% if baseline < 3 μg/L/hr (ng/cc/hr)

REFERENCES

1. Slataper RM, Bakris GL: Secondary hypertension. In Taylor R (ed): Difficult Diagnosis II. Philadelphia, W.B. Saunders, 1992, pp 403–411.
2. Rudnick MR, Maxwell MH: Limitations of renin assays. In Narins RG (ed): Controversies in Nephrology and Hypertension. New York, Churchill-Livingstone, 1984, pp 123–160.
3. McCarthy JE, Weder AB: The captopril test and renovascular hypertension: A cautionary tale. Arch Intern Med 1990;150:493–495.
4. Setaro JF, Saddler MC, Chen CC, et al: Simplified captopril renography in the diagnosis and treatment of renal artery stenosis. Hypertension 1991;18:289–298.
5. Davidson R, Wilcox CS: Diagnostic usefulness of renal scanning after angiotensin converting enzyme inhibitors [editorial]. Hypertension 1991;18:299–303.
6. Black HR, Nally JV (eds): The role of captopril scintography in the diagnosis and management of renovascular hypertension: A consensus conference. Am J Hypertens 1991;4(suppl):661S–751S.
7. Setaro JF, Chen CC, Hoffer PB, Black HR: Captopril renography in the diagnosis of renal artery stenosis and the prediction of improvement with revascularization: The Yale Vascular Center experience. Am J Hypertens 1991;4(suppl):698S–705S.
8. Black HR: Captopril renal scintography—A way to distinguish functional from anatomic renal artery stenosis. J Nucl Med 1992;33:2045–2046.

APPENDIX V

Medications Commonly Used in the Treatment of Hypertension

APPENDIX V

Medications Commonly Used in the Treatment of Hypertension

Medication		Dosage			Side Effects		Availability		
Class/Drug	Brand Names	Start Dose	Adjustment Intervals	Maximum Dosage	Frequent	Infrequent	Dose Sizes	Tablet or Capsule	Scored
Thiazide diuretics									
Hydrochloro-thiazide	HydroDiuril and others	12.5 mg once daily	2–3 weeks	25 mg/day*	Impotence Hypokalemia Hypomagnesemia Hyperuricemia Hyperglycemia Hyperlipidemia (transient) Mild metabolic alkalosis Hyponatremia Ineffective in renal failure (except metolazone)	Acute interstitial nephritis Blood dyscrasias Rash	25,50,100 mg	Tab	Yes
Indapamide	Lozol	1.25–2.5 mg once daily	2 weeks	2.5 mg/day	Same as thiazides without hyperlipidemia	Same as other thiazides	1.25,2.5 mg	Tab	No
Metolazone	Diulo Zaroxolyn	1.25 mg once daily	2 weeks	10 mg/day	Same as other thiazides but effective in renal failure	Same as other thiazides	2.5,5,10 mg	Tab	No
Loop diuretics									
Furosemide	Lasix	20 mg twice daily	2 weeks	600 mg/day	Impotence Hypokalemia Hypomagnesemia Hyperuricemia Hyperglycemia Hyperlipidemia Metabolic alkalosis Hypernatremia	Hyponatremia Hypocalcemia Blood dyscrasia Rash Acute interstitial nephritis Thromboembolism	20,40,80 mg	Tab	Yes (except 20 mg)
Ethacrynic acid	Edecrin	12.5 mg twice daily	3 weeks	400 mg/day	Same as furosemide	Same as furosemide	25,50 mg	Tab	Yes

Butmetanide	Bumex	0.25 mg twice daily	3 weeks	10 mg/day	Same as furosemide	Same as furosemide	0.5,1,2 mg	Tab	No
Torsemide	Demadex	2.5 mg daily	3 weeks(?)	200 mg/day	Same as furosemide	Same as furosemide	5,10,20,100 mg	Tab	Yes
Potassium-sparing diuretics (Main use to prevent or correct hypokalemia)									
Spironolactone	Aldactone	25 mg once daily	—	400 mg/day	Hyperkalemia Gastrointestinal disturbances Gynecomastia	Rash Hyponatremia Agranulocytosis	25,50,100 mg	Tab	Only 100s
Triamterene	Dyrenium	50 mg once daily	—	200 mg/day	Hyperkalemia Gastrointestinal disturbances Not antihypertensive	Triamterene kidney stones	50,100 mg	Tab	No
Amiloride	Midamor	5 mg once daily	—	10 mg/day[†]	Hyperkalemia Gastrointestinal disturbances Headache	Rash	5 mg	Tab	No
Central alpha-2 agonists									
Clonidine	Catapres	0.1 mg once or twice daily	3 days	2.4 mg/day	Dry mouth Urinary retention Somnolence	Sodium retention Insomnia	0.1,0.2,0.3 mg	Tab	No
	Catapres-TTS patches	2.5 mg every week	2 weeks	15 mg (2 TTS-3 patches) weekly	Worsening AV block Bradycardia Fatigue Rash with patches		TTS:2.5,5, 7.5 mg	Patch	—
Methyldopa	Aldomet	250 mg twice daily	3 days	2000 mg/day	Somnolence Worsening AV block Bradycardia Fatigue Orthostasis Positive Coomb's test[‡]	Hepatitis[‡] Hemolysis	125,250, 500 mg	Tab	No
Guanabenz	Wytensin	4 mg twice daily	—	16 mg/day	Same as clonidine	Same as clonidine	4,8,16 mg	Tab	No
Guanfacine	Tenex	1 mg once daily at bedtime	3 weeks	3 mg/day	Same as clonidine	Same as clonidine	1,2 mg	Tab	No

Continued on following page.

Medications Commonly Used in the Treatment of Hypertension *(Continued)*

Medication		Dosage			Side Effects		Availability		
Class/Drug	Brand Names	Start Dose	Adjustment Intervals	Maximum Dosage	Frequent	Infrequent	Dose Sizes	Tablet or Capsule	Scored
Peripheral alpha-1 blockers (Arteriolar and venous dilators)									
Prazosin	Minipress	1 mg at bedtime, then twice daily	2 weeks	20 mg/day	First-dose orthostasis Dizziness Fatigue Headache Somnolence	Leukopenia	1,2,5 mg	Cap	No
Terazosin	Hytrin	Same as prazosin, but once daily	2 weeks	20 mg/day	Same as prazosin	Same as prazosin	1,2,5,10 mg	Cap	No
Doxazosin	Cardura	Same as prazosin, but once daily	2 weeks	16 mg/day	Same as prazosin	Same as prazosin	1,2,4,8 mg	Tab	Yes
Nonselective beta blockers without ISA§									
Propranolol	Inderal Inderal-LA	20 mg two or three times daily LA 80 mg once or twice daily	2–4 weeks	1000 mg/day	Fatigue Exacerbation of asthma Masking of hyperglycemia Delay of recovery from hypoglycemia Worsening of hypertension during hypoglycemia Impotence Worsening of Raynaud's Worsening of arterial insufficiency(?) Reduction of renal blood flow Negative inotropic and chronotropic effects Worsening of hyperlipidemia		10,20,30,40 80 mg LA: 80,120, 160 mg	Tab	Yes

Nadolol	Corgard	40 mg once daily	2–4 weeks	480 mg/day	Same as propranolol	20,40,80,120, 160 mg	Tab	Yes
Timolol	Blocadren	10 mg twice daily	2–4 weeks	60 mg/day	Same as propranolol	5,10,20 mg	Tab	Yes (except 5 mg)
Nonselective beta blockers with ISA§ (Preferred for patients with symptomatic bradycardia; do not affect serum lipids; may not reduce mortality after myocardial infarction as with non-ISA drugs.)								
Pindolol	Visken	5 mg twice daily	2–4 weeks	60 mg/day	Like propranolol, except Less chronotropic effect Preserves renal blood flow No adverse effects on lipids	5,10 mg	Tab	No
Penbutolol	Levatol	10 mg once daily	2–4 weeks	20 mg/day	Same as pindolol	20 mg	Long Tab	No
Beta-1 selective blockers without ISA (Selective only in low doses; may be preferred for diabetics since these may not delay recovery from hypoglycemia and are less likely to exacerbate hypertension during hypoglycemia.)								
Atenolol	Tenormin	50 mg once daily	2–4 weeks	100 mg/day	In low dose: Fatigue Depression Impotence Negative chronotropic and inotropic effects In higher doses: All of nonselective effects (like propranolol, including lowering high-density lipoproteins	25,50,100 mg	Tab	Only 50 mg
Metoprolol	Lopressor	50 mg twice daily	2–4 weeks	400 mg/day	Like atenolol *plus* elevates blood levels of verapamil	50,100 mg	Long Tab	No
	Toprol XL	25–50 mg once daily				50,100,200	Tab	Yes

Continued on following page.

Medications Commonly Used in the Treatment of Hypertension *(Continued)*

Medication		Dosage			Side Effects		Availability		
Class/Drug	Brand Names	Start Dose	Adjustment Intervals	Maximum Dosage	Frequent	Infrequent	Dose Sizes	Tablet or Capsule	Scored
Beta-1 selective blockers without ISA *(Cont.)*									
Betaxolol	Kerlone	5–10 mg once daily	2–4 weeks	20 mg/day	Like metoprolol *plus* headache, but no adverse effect on high-density lipoproteins		10,20 mg	Tab	Only 10 mg
Beta-1 selective blocker with ISA									
Acebutolol	Sectral	200 mg once daily	2–4 weeks	600 mg/day	Fatigue Depression Impotence Loses beta-1 selectivity at higher doses	—	200,400 mg	Cap	No
Combined alpha-1 and beta blocker with ISA									
Labetalol	Trandate Normodyne	200 mg twice daily	3 days	2400 mg/ day(?)	Bronchospasm Fatigue Severe orthostasis Impotence Paresthesias Nonselective at higher doses	Hepatitis Lupus Tremor	100,200, 300 mg	Cap	No
Nondihydropyridine calcium channel blockers									
Diltiazem	Cardizem	30 mg three times daily	4 weeks	540 mg/day	Moderately negative inotropic effects	—	30,60,90 120 mg	Cap	
	Cardizem SR	60 mg twice daily			Mild SA and AV conduction disturbances		60,90,120 mg	Cap	
	Cardizem CD	180 mg once daily			Increased digoxin levels Constipation		180,240, 300 mg	Cap	
	Dilacor XR	180 mg once daily			Mild edema Use beta blocker with caution				

Verapamil	Calan	40 mg three times daily	4 weeks	480 mg/day	Most negatively inotropic effects Greatest AV block Most constipating	Gingival hyperplasia	40,80,120 mg	Tab	Yes (except 40 mg)
	Calan SR	120 mg once or twice daily					120,180, 249 mg	Tab	Yes (except 120 mg)
	Verelan	120 mg once or twice daily					120,180, 240 mg	Cap	No
	Isoptin						40,80,120 mg	Tab	Yes
	Isoptin SR						120,180, 240 mg	Tab	Yes (except 120 mg)
Dihydropyridine calcium channel blockers									
Nifedipine	Procardia Adalat	10 mg three times daily	4 weeks	120 mg/day	Tachycardia Headache Local edema Orthostasis Mildly negative inotropic effects Flushing	Gingival hyperplasia	10,20 mg	Cap	No
	Procardia XL Adalat CC	30 mg once daily					30,60,90 mg	Tab	No
Nicardipine	Cardene	20 mg three times daily	4 weeks	120 mg/day	Tachycardia Local edema Headache	Gingival hyperplasia	20,30 mg	Cap	No
	Cardene SR	30 mg twice daily					30,45,60 mg	Cap	No
Felodipine	Plendil	5 mg once daily	3 weeks	20 mg/day	Same as nicardipine	—	2.5,10 mg	Tab	No
Amlodipine	Norvasc	2.5 mg once daily	3 weeks	10 mg/day	Same as nicardipine	—	2.5,5,10 mg	Tab	No
Isradipine	DynaCirc	2.5 mg twice daily	4 weeks	10 mg/day	Same as nicardipine		2.5,5 mg	Cap	No
Bepridil	Vascor	200 mg once daily	10 days	400 mg/day	Same as nicardipine		200,300, 400 mg	Tab	No

Continued on following page.

Medications Commonly Used in the Treatment of Hypertension *(Continued)*

Medication		Dosage			Side Effects		Availability		
Class/Drug	Brand Names	Start Dose	Adjustment Intervals	Maximum Dosage	Frequent	Infrequent	Dose Sizes	Tablet or Capsule	Scored
Direct-acting vasodilators									
Hydralazine	Apresoline	10–20 mg two to four times daily	1 week	300–400 mg/day	Tachycardia[‖] Fluid retention Angina Headache Positive antinuclear antibodies	Lupus Nasal congestion Rash Hepatitis Glomerulonephritis	10,25,50, 100 mg	Tab	No
Minoxidil	Loniten	5 mg once daily	4 days	80 mg/day	Tachycardia[‖] Fluid retention Angina Hypertrichosis Coarse facial features (like acromegaly)	Pericardial effusion Hemopericardium Pulmonary fibrosis Cytopenias	2,5,10 mg	Tab	Yes
Angiotensin converting enzyme inhibitors									
Captopril	Capoten Capoten-LA	12.5 mg two or three times daily	2 weeks	150 mg/day	Cough Flushing Hyperkalemia Dysgeusia Orthostasis	Azotemia Angioedema Cytopenias Erythroderma Membranous nephropathy	12.5,25,37.5, 50,100 mg	Tab	Only 12.5 mg
Enalapril	Vasotec	2.5 mg once or twice daily	1–2 weeks	60–80 mg/day	Same as captopril	Same as captopril	2.5,5,10,20 mg	Tab	Only 2.5 and 5 mg
Lisinopril	Zestril Prinivil	10 mg once daily or 5 mg twice daily	2–4 weeks	60–80 mg/day	Same as captopril	Same as captopril	5,10,20,40 mg	Tab	Only 5 mg
Ramipril	Altace	1.25–2.5 mg once or twice daily	2–4 weeks	40 mg/day	Same as captopril	Same as captopril	1.25,2.5,5, 10 mg	Cap	No
Benzapril	Lotensin	5–10 mg once or twice daily	2–4 weeks	40–80 mg/day	Same as captopril	Same as captopril	5,10,20,40 mg	Tab	No
Fosinopril	Monopril	10 mg once or twice daily	2–4 weeks	80 mg/ day	Same as captopril	Same as captopril	10,20 mg	Tab	No
Quinapril	Accupril	10 mg once daily or 5 mg twice daily	2–4 weeks	80 mg/day	Same as captopril	Same as captopril	5,10,20,40 mg	Tab	Yes

Angiotensin II receptor antagonist									
Losartan	Cozaar	25–50 mg	3–6 weeks	100 mg/day	Muscle cramps, backache, postural hypotension, nasal congestion, probably azotemia in patients with congestive heart failure or renal artery stenosis or in some patients with preexisting nephrosclerosis	Hyperkalemia, angioedema, serious dermatologic reactions, abnormal liver function tests	25,50 mg	Tab	No
Postganglionic agents									
Guanethidine	Ismelin	10 mg once daily	1–2 weeks	300 mg/day	Diarrhea, postural hypotension, syncope, fluid retention, nausea and vomiting, dry mouth, blurred vision, fatigue, depression, impaired ejaculation, precipitation of asthma, edema, angina, urinary incontinence, nocturia, nasal stuffiness	Parotid gland tenderness, congestive heart failure, ptosis, myalgia, dermatitis, alopecia, blood dyscrasia, priapism, azotemia	10,25 mg	Tab	Yes
Guanadrel	Hylorel	5 mg twice daily	1 week	150 mg/day	Same as guanethidine ? less severe	Same as guanethidine	10,25 mg	Tab	Yes
Reserpine	Serpasil	0.05 mg once daily	3 weeks	1 mg/day	Depression, drowsiness, nasal congestion, weight gain, abdominal cramps, diarrhea, fluid retention, dyspepsia, exacerbation of peptic ulcer, impotence, bronchospasm	Extrapyramidal effects	0.1, 0.25 mg	Tab	No

* Although higher doses may be needed in other diseases (e.g., nephrolithiasis), doses higher than 25 mg/day add only slightly to control of hypertension.

† Except in patients with primary hyperaldosteronism, who may need 40 mg/day (*see* chapter 4).

‡ Stop methyldopa for abnormal liver function or hemolytic anemia, but not just for positive Coombs' test.

§ ISA = intrinsic sympathomimetic activity.

// The common adverse effects of tachycardia, angina, and fluid retention seen with either hydralazine or minoxidil, usually are largely preventable through the concurrent use of diuretics and either beta blockers or central agents.

APPENDIX V
(Supplement)

Common Combination Antihypertensive Drugs*

Medication		Availability		
Class/Drug*	Brand Names	Dose Sizes	Tablet or Capsule	Scored
Combination diuretics				
Hydrochlorothiazide/spironolactone†	Aldactazide	25/25 mg 50/50 mg	Tab Tab	No Yes
Hydrochlorothiazide/triamterene†	Dyazide Maxzide-25 Maxzide	25/37.5 mg 25/37.5 mg 50/75 mg	Cap Tab Tab	No Yes Yes
Hydrochlorothiazide/amiloride†	Moduretic	50/5 mgm	Tab	Yes
Diuretic/nonselective beta blockers				
Hydrochlorothiazide/propranolol†	Inderide Inderide-LA	25/40 & 25/80 mg 50/80, 50/120, & 50/160 mg	Tab Cap	Yes No
Hydrochlorothiazide/timolol	Timolide	25/10 mg	Tab	No
Diuretic/selective beta-1 blockers				
Chlorthalidone/atenolol	Tenoretic	20/50 & 25/100 mg	Tab	Yes (only 25/50)
Hydrochlorothiazide/bisoprolol	Ziac	6.25/2.5, 6.25/5, 6.25/10 mg	Tab	No
Hydrochlorothiazide/metoprolol	Lopressor HCT	25/50, 25/100 & 50/100 mg	Long Tab	Yes
Diuretic/alpha-2 blocker				
Polythiazide/prazosin	Minizide	0.5/1, 0.5/2, 0.5/5 mg	Cap	No
Diuretic/ACE inhibitors				
Hydrochlorothiazide/captopril	Capozide	25/15, 25/25, 50/15 & 50/50 mg	Tab	No
Hydrochlorothiazide/enalapril	Vaseretic	25/10 mg	Tab	No
Hydrochlorothiazide/lisinopril	Zestoretic Prinzide	12.5/20 & 25/20 mg	Tab	No
Hydrochlorothiazide/benazepril	Lotensin HCT	6.2/5, 12.5/10, 12.5/20,25/20	Tab	Yes
Diuretic/central agents				
Hydrochlorothiazide/methyldopa†	Aldoril	15/250, 25/250, 30/500 & 50/500 mg	Tab	No
Chlorothiazide/methyldopa	Aldoclor	150/250 & 250/250 mg	Tab	No
Chlorthalidone/clonidine†	Combipres	15/0.1, 15/0.2, & 15/0.3 mg	Tab	Yes
Diuretic/vasodilator				
Hydrochlorothiazide/hydralazine	Apresazide	25/25, 50/50, & 50/100 mg	Cap	No

Continued on following page.

Common Combination Antihypertensive Drugs*

Medication		Availability		
Class/Drug*	Brand Names	Dose Sizes	Tablet or Capsule	Scored
Diuretic/postganglionic inhibitors				
Chlorthalidone/reserpine	Regroton Demi-regroton	50/0.25 mg 25/0.25 mg	Tab	No
Chlorothiazide/reserpine†	Diupress	250/0.125 mg, 500/0.125 mg	Tab	Yes
Hydrochlorothiazide/reserpine†	Hydropress	25/0.125 mg, 50/0.125 mg	Tab	Yes
Hydroflumethiazide/reserpine†	Salutensin-demi Salutensin	25/0.125 mg 50/0.125 mg	Tab	No
Hydrochlorothiazide/guanethidine	Esimil	25/100 mg	Tab	Yes
Diuretic/vasodilator/postganglionic inhibitor				
Hydrochlorothiazide/hydralazine/reserpine	Ser-Ap-Es	15/25/0.1 mg	Tab	No
Diuretic/angiotensin II blocker				
Hydrochlorothiazide/losartan	Hyzaar	12.5/50 mg	Tab	No

*Note: Combination drugs may increase compliance, but generally should be reserved for selected patients. Generally, patients should be titrated on uncombined drugs. When the final dosage is reached, if a suitable combination drug *with the same dosages* is available, it may be substituted. Combinations of thiazide and potassium-retaining diuretics should generally be avoided in diabetic or other patients prone to hyperkalemia; the thiazide-ACE inhibitor combinations may be useful in diabetic or other patients who are *mildly* hyperkalemic on ACE inhibitors alone (potassium prior to addition of diuretics, but after ACE inhibitors *below 6.0*). Patients with severe hyperkalemia after the addition of ACE inhibitors (potassium of 6.0 or greater) should generally not recieve them, even with thiazide diuretics. Generally, the drugs with the lowest possible doses of diuretic are preferred, and doses of thiazides for the treatment of hypertension should be below 50 mg/day. Also note that several ACE inhibitor/calcium channel blocker combinations were in development at the time of this writing.

†Denotes combination drugs available as generic.

APPENDIX VI

Dosage Adjustments in Renal Impairment

APPENDIX VI

Dosage Adjustments in Renal Impairment

I. **Medications which usually do not require adjustment with renal insufficiency**
  A. Diuretics
    1. Furosemide
    2. Metolazone
    3. Bumetanide
  B. Central agents
    1. Clonidine
    2. Guanabenz
    3. Guanfacine
  C. Alpha blockers
    1. Prazosin
    2. Doxazosin
    3. Terazosin
  D. Beta blockers (Use beta blockers and/or ACE inhibitors in renal failure with extreme caution, especially in combination, because of the danger of hyperkalemia.)
    1. Nonselective without intrinsic sympathomimetic activity (ISA)
      a. Propranolol
      b. Timolol
    2. Beta-1 selective without ISA
      a. Metoprolol
    3. Nonselective with ISA
      a. Penbutolol
      b. Pindolol
    4. Combined beta-1 and alpha blocker
      a. Labetalol
  E. Angiotensin-converting enzyme inhibitors (Use beta blockers and/or ACE inhibitors in renal failure with extreme caution, especially in combination, because of the danger of hyperkalemia.)
    1. Fosinopril
  F. Direct vasodilators
    1. Minoxidil
  G. Calcium channel blockers
    1. All
  H. Nitrates
    1. All

II. **Drugs generally contraindicated or ineffective in renal failure**
  A. All potassium-conserving diuretics
  B. Acetazolamide
  C. Indapamide
  D. Thiazides (except metolazone)
  E. Reserpine

III. **Drugs to be used only with caution in renal impairment**
  A. Beta blockers and ACE inhibitors
    1. Monitor renal function and potassium closely.
    2. Discontinue if possible if hyperkalemia is significant.

3. ACE inhibitors are contraindicated in anyone with a history of hyperkalemia, or with patients on other drugs that may raise serum potassium (*see* Appendix VIII).

B. Nitroprusside
   1. Although dosage is unchanged, toxic metabolites accumulate sooner.
   2. Monitor levels of thiocyanate closely if using for more than 24–48 hours.

C. Nonselective beta blockers without ISA
   1. Significant risk of prolonged hypoglycemia in diabetics
   2. Significant risk of spontaneous or worsened hyperkalemia
   3. Can reduce renal blood flow.

D. Methyldopa
   1. Long-acting metabolites persist for days.
   2. Orthostatic hypotension limits usefulness, especially in uremia.

REFERENCES

1. Bennett WM. Practical guidelines for drug dosing in renal failure. In Bennett WM, McCarron DA (eds): Contemporary Issues in Nephrology, vol. 17. New York, Churchill-Livingstone, 1987, pp 352–387.
2. Bakris GL: Drug dosages for patients with renal failure. In Stein JH: Internal Medicine: Diagnosis and Therapy, 3rd ed. Norwalk, Appleton & Croft, 1993, pp 352–387.
3. Bennett WM, Aronoff GR, Golper TA, et al: Drug Prescribing in Renal Failure. Philadelphia, American College of Physicians, 1987.
4. Schrier RW, Gambertoglio JG (eds): Handbook of Drug Therapy in Liver and Kidney Disease. Boston, Little Brown, 1991.

APPENDIX VII

Side Effects of Antihypertensive Medications

APPENDIX VII

Side Effects of Antihypertensive Medications

TABLE A14. Relatively Benign and Non-Life-Threatening Drug Reactions

Symptom or Conditions	Drugs Possibly Beneficial	Drugs Possibly Harmful
Headache	Calcium blockers Central agents Beta blockers	Hydralazine Alpha blockers Calcium blockers
Hot flashes	Clonidine	Calcium blockers
Anxiety	Beta blockers Central agents Reserpine	—
Lethargy	—	Central agents Beta blockers
Impotence	ACE inhibitors	All except ACE inhibitors
Constipation	Guanethidine	Calcium blockers Diuretics Central agents Trimethaphan
Diarrhea	Calcium blockers Diuretics Central agents	Reserpine Guanethidine
Essential tremor	Beta blockers	—
Baldness	Minoxidil	Hydralazine
Rhinorrhea or tearing	Clonidine	Beta blockers
Edema	Diuretics Beta blockers (?)	Alpha blockers Calcium blockers Hydralazine Minoxidil Methyldopa
Insomnia	Central agents	—

TABLE A15. Potentially Serious Adverse Drug Reactions

Conditions or Symptom	Drugs Possibly Beneficial	Drugs Possibly Harmful	Contraindicated
Isolated systolic hypertension	Long-acting nitrates Beta blockers Alpha blockers Diuretics Calcium blockers	—	—
Asthma	Dihydropyridine Calcium blockers	High-dose diuretics ACE inhibitors All alpha agents	Beta blockers (all)
Diabetes	ACE inhibitors* Heart-rate-lowering calcium channel blockers	High-dose diuretics Beta-1 selective blockers	Beta blockers (nonselective)

Continued on following page.

TABLE A15. Potentially Serious Adverse Drug Reactions *(Continued)*

Conditions or Symptom	Drugs Possibly Beneficial	Drugs Possibly Harmful	Contraindicated
Tachyarrhythmias	Beta blockers Heart-rate-lowering calcium channel blockers Central agents	Hydralazine[†] Nifedipine[†]	—
Bradyarrhythmias	Hydralazine	Central agents Beta blockers	—
Renal insufficiency	ACE inhibitors* Calcium channel blockers Alpha blockers Metolazone Loop diuretics	Ace inhibitors Beta blockers (especially non-selective) Nitroprusside Diazoxide	Thiazides (except metolazone)
Bilateral renal artery stenosis or solitary kidney	Calcium blockers (?) Beta blockers	ACE inhibitors	—
Left ventricular hypertrophy	Calcium blockers Beta blockers Central agents Diuretics[2] Ace inhibitors[3]	—	—
Hyperlipidemia	Alpha blockers Calcium blockers	Beta blocker[‡] without ISA Diuretics[§]	—
Hyperkalemia	Diuretics (not potassium-retaining)	Calcium channel blockers[¶] Beta blockers	Potassium-retaining diuretics ACE inhibitors
Depression	—	Beta blockers Reserpine Central alpha agonists (antagonized by tricyclics) ACE inhibitors if on lithium	Diuretics if on lithium
Angina	Beta blockers Calcium blockers	Diuretics	Hydralazine (without beta blockade) Guanethidine Minoxidil (without beta blockade)
Congestive heart failure	Diuretics Ace inhibitors Amlodipine (?)	Beta blockers Diltiazem Other calcium blockers	Verapamil
Post-myocardial infarction	Beta blockers (without ISA) Heart-rate-lowering calcium channel blockers	Hydralazine	—

Continued on following page.

TABLE A15. Potentially Serious Adverse Drug Reactions *(Continued)*

Conditions or Symptom	Drugs Possibly Beneficial	Drugs Possibly Harmful	Contraindicated
Orthostasis or cerebral ischemia	Beta blockers Clonidine	Labetalol Guanethidine Diuretics Methyldopa ACE inhibitors (especially with diuretics)	—
Pregnancy	Methyldopa	Some beta blockers (?) Diuretics	ACE inhibitors Nitroprusside (avoid if possible)
Pheochromocytoma	Peripheral alpha blockers Heart-rate-lowering calcium channel blockers	—	Minoxidil Beta blocker without alpha blockade
AV block or bradycardia	Hydralazine	Guanethidine Central agents Reserpine	Beta blockers Verapamil Diltiazem
Liver disease	—	Methyldopa Labetalol Hydralazine	—
Systemic lupus erythematosus	—	—	Hydralazine Methyldopa Acebutolol

* Ace inhibitors and calcium channel blockers (or both together) slow the progression of *early* diabetic renal disease, but both (particularly ACE inhibitors) can worsen renal disease under certain circumstances (*see* Chapter 4). There is a significant risk of serious hyperkalemia in patients with renal impairment, especially diabetics in whom ACE inhibitors are used. Twenty-four hour urine protein determinations *must* be obtained prior to and during the use of ACE inhibitors in these patients. Serum creatinine should also be checked during the first week of therapy and frequently thereafter.

† Reflex tachycardia is common.

‡ Beta blockers with ISA (intrinsic sympathomimetic activity) and at least one beta-1 selective blocker (betaxolol) do not seem to adversely affect lipid profiles.

§ Worsening or new onset of hyperlipidemia may not occur with certain diuretics and often is transient when it does occur. In some cases, alpha blockers have been reported to reverse elevations in lipids accompanying drug usage.

¶ Directly inhibit aldosterone release.

REFERENCES

1. SHEP Cooperative Research Group: Prevention of stroke by antihypertensive drug treatment in older persons with isolated systolic hypertension. JAMA 1991;265:3255–3264.
2. Neaton JD, Grimm RH, Prineas RJ, et al: Treatment of mild hypertension study: Final results. JAMA 1993;270:713–724.
3. Frohlich ED, Horinaka S: Cardiac and aortic effects of angiotensin converting enzyme inhibitors. Hypertension 1991;18(suppl II):II2–II7..

APPENDIX VIII

Important Drug Interactions

APPENDIX VIII

Important Drug Interactions*

Drug	Second Drug	Reaction	Comments
Beta blockers or Labetalol	Central alpha agent (e.g., methyldopa, clonidine)	Severe paradoxical hypertension	Taper other to zero by 3 days prior to new drug. Avoid concurrent use; should not be used in combination. No additional pressure lowering.
	Peripheral alpha blocker	Exaggerated first-dose orthostasis	Lower initial dose.
	Calcium blocker	Conduction defects	Less with dihydropyridine (nifedipine, etc.).
	Hydralazine	Increased beta blockade	
	Thiazides	Greater hyperglycemia	More severe with hypokalemia.
	NSAIDs[†]	Impaired antihypertensive effect	Avoid this class.
		Hyperkalemia	Especially if renal insufficiency or other interacting drugs are present.
		Worsening renal function	Avoid this combination in renal impairment.
	ACE inhibitors	Hyperkalemia	Monitor potassium levels, especially in diabetics.
	OTC adrenergic agonists	Hypertension	Due to unopposed alpha activity; avoid.
Calcium blocker	Peripheral alpha blocker	Hypotension	Use with care; avoid nifedipine.
	Beta blockers	Congestive heart failure, conduction disturbances	Least for nifedipine.
	Carbamazepine, rifampin, or phenobarbital	Decrease blood levels of calcium blockers	—
	Cyclosporine	Increased cyclosporine levels (only with nondihydropyridines)	Watch levels closely if on verapamil or diltiazem
	Magnesium sulfate	Neuromuscular blockade Hypotension	Combination of these two drugs to treat preeclampsia is under study.
ACE inhibitors	Lithium	High serum lithium levels	Use with extreme caution; monitor levels.
	Diuretics	Hypotension	Taper off diuretics prior to using, or use tiny doses initially.
		Worsening renal function	Avoid this combination with renal artery stenosis.

Continued on following page.

Important Drug Interactions* *(Continued)*

Drug	Second Drug	Reaction	Comments
ACE inhibitors *(Cont.)*	Potassium-sparing diuretics	Hyperkalemia, especially with spironolactone	Avoid combination.
	Beta-blockers	Hyperkalemia	Monitor potassium levels, especially in diabetics.
	NSAIDs†	Hyperkalemia Renal insufficiency	Monitor potassium levels, especially in diabetics. Contraindicated combination (avoid this combination, *especially* with renal impairment or hepatic dysfunction).
	Antacids	Decreased bioavailability	—
Methyldopa	Oral iron	Decreased methyldopa absorption	—
	Lithium	May increase lithium levels	—
	Tricyclic antidepressants	May antagonize antihypertensive effect	—
	Trifluoperazine	Severe hypertension	Prolongs half-life of catecholamines; avoid.
Clonidine	Monoamine oxidase inhibitors	Hallucinations	Avoid concurrent use if possible.
	Haloperidol	Dementia	Stop both drugs if it occurs.
	Diazoxide	Severe hypotension	Avoid concurrent use.
	NSAIDs†	Impaired antihypertensive effect	Avoid if possible.
	Tricyclic antidepressants	May antagonize antihypertensive effect	—
Alpha blockers	NSAIDs†	Impaired antihypertensive effect.	Avoid if possible.

Additional interactions reported to result in severe hypertension

Combination of amitriptyline, sinemet, and metoclopramide[4]

Combination of doxepin, chlorpromazine, and guanethidine[5];

Levodopa (without carbidopa) and selegiline (or other monoamine oxidase inhibitors)[6–8];

Guanadrel, buspirone, and amantadine have all been reported to cause increased hypertension with monoamine oxidase inhibitors.

* There are many potential drug interactions which are not listed here; one should always consult a drug interaction handbook or (preferably) a computerized interaction database[1] when scrutinizing medications in a hypertensive patient. OTC = over the counter.

† Impaired antihypertensive efficacy of all drugs except calcium blockers reported for patients on most NSAIDs (nonsteroidal antiinflammatory drugs).

REFERENCES

1. Rizack MA, Hillman CDM: The Medical Letter Drug Interaction Program for the IBM-PC. New Rochelle, NY, The Medical Letter, 1993.
2. Rizack MA, Hillman CDM: The Medical Letter Handbook of Adverse Drug Interactions. New Rochelle, NY, The Medical Letter, 1993.
3. Campbell N, Paddock V, Sundaram R: Alteration of methyldopa absorption, metabolism, and blood pressure control caused by ferrous sulfate and ferrous gluconate. Clin Pharmacol Ther 1988;43:381.
4. Rampton DS: Hypertensive crisis in a patient given Sinemet, metoclopramide, and amitriptyline. BMJ 1977;1977;2:607–608.
5. Poe TE, Edwards JL, Taylor RB: Hypertensive crisis possibly due to a drug interaction. Postgrad Med 1979;66:235–347.
6. Schildkraut JJ, et al: Biochemical and pressor effects of oral D,L-dihydroxyphenylalanine in patients pretreated with antidepressant drugs. Ann NY Acad Sci 1963;107:1005.
7. Hunter KR: Monoamine oxidase inhibitors and L-dopa. BMJ 1970;3:388.
8. Baronti F, et al: Deprenyl effects on levodopa pharmacodynamics, mood, and free radical scavenging. Neurology 1992;42:541.

APPENDIX IX

Parenteral Medications Used in the Treatment of Hypertension

APPENDIX IX

Parenteral Medications Used in the Treatment of Hypertension[1,2,3,4]

Medication		Dosage			Indications and Side Effects	
Class/Drug (Brand Name)	Onset	Starting Dose*/Drip	Adjustment Interval and Usual Dose	Maximum Doses	Indications or Use	Side Effects†
Diuretics						
Furosemide (Lasix)	15–60 min	20–80 mg intravenously	Usually 1–2 hr	600 mg/day or dose; give no faster than 20 mg/min when giving doses over 80 mg intravenously.	Congestive heart failure (*not* for other hypertensive emergencies)	Deafness when given quickly
Ethacrynic acid (Edecrin)	5 min	25 mg intravenously, *slowly*	Variable, usually 1–2 hr	100-mg dose; slow push or by infusion.	Congestive heart failure (*not* for other hyper tensive emergencies)	Deafness when given quickly Phlebitis—avoid repeated injection in same peripheral site.
Beta blockers						
Propranolol (Inderal)	≤ 5 min	0.5 mg Do not exceed 1-mg/min injection rate.	1 mg every 5 min until pulse pressure is < 60 mmHg or 0.15 mg/kg (10 mg) or significant bradyarrhythmia or heart block. Then 0.5–2 mg every 4–6 hr.	Guided by response	Aortic dissection (with nitroprusside)	Hypotension Bradycardia Bronchospasm Requires constant ECG monitoring, especially during administration.
Metoprolol (Lopressor)	20 min	5 mg every 2 min to max of 15 mg	Repeat every 6 hr	60 mg	Pregnancy Aortic dissection (?)	Same as propranolol
Esmolol (Breviblock)	5 min	*Load:* 0.5 mg/kg over 1 min *Drip:* 0.05 mg/kg/min to start after	Repeat loading dose every 5 min as needed, while adjusting drip up, in 0.05-mg/kg/min increments.	0.3 mg/kg/min	Beta-1 blockade after alpha blockade in operating room for excessive beta activity when removing a pheochromocytoma.	Same as propranolol

Calcium channel blockers						
Nicardipine (Cardene I.V.)	Minutes	*Drip:* 0.1 mg/ml Start 50 cc/hr (5 mg/hr) Increase by 25 cc/hr every 15 min as needed.	Increase by 25 ml/hr (2.5 mg/hr) every 15 min Once controlled, reduce to 20 ml/hr, then titrate as needed.	Maximum of 150 ml/hr (15 mg/hr)	Maintenance in N.P.O. patients. May be used in heart failure and coronary artery disease. May improve cardiac output in some patients with heart failure. Usually improves coronary blood flow.	Takes 45 min or more to reach steady state; takes 30 min or more for effects to wane; lowers pressure more in hypertensive patients. Tachycardia may occur. Avoid with aortic stenosis or patients on cyclosporine. Can have negative inotropic effects, especially with beta blockers.
Combined alpha and beta blocker						
Labetalol (Normodyne, Trandate)	5 min (bolus)	*Bolus:* 20 mg intravenously *Infusion:* 800 mg/250 ml fluid (only after bolus)	*Bolus:* every 10 min to max of 300 mg *Infusion:* (after initial bolus) of 1–2 mg/min *Adjust* drip every 4–8 hr (long half-life) or discontinue for hypotension)	300-mg boluses or 2400 mg/day infused	Early myocardial infarction Malignant hypertension Aortic dissection	Postural hypotension
Central alpha agonists						
Methyldopa (Aldomet)	4–6 hr	125–250 mg	125–500 mg every 4–12 hr	2000 mg/day	Intravenous maintenance or urgent therapy in patients unable to take oral medicine or be tube fed.	—

Continued on following page.

Parenteral Medications Used in the Treatment of Hypertension *(Continued)*

Medication			Dosage		Indications and Side Effects	
Class/Drug (Brand Name)	Onset	Starting Dose*/Drip	Adjustment Interval and Usual Dose	Maximum Doses	Indications or Use	Side Effects[†]
Direct arteriolar vasodilators						
Hydralazine (Apresoline)	10 min intravenously	5 mg	5–20 mg intravenously (or up to 50 mg intramuscularly if necessary) every 30 min	200 mg/day	Preeclampsia/eclampsia	Headache Tachycardia Neonatal thrombocytopenia Angina
Diazoxide (Hyperstat)	5–15 min	30 mg *Drip:* 7.5–30 mg/min	30–150 mg every 5 min initially	5 mg/kg	Preeclampsia, eclampsia	Fluid retention Tachycardia Hyperglycemia Dyspnea Cough Phlebitis (avoid nonintravenous administration) Angina Transient cerebrovascular ischemic attacks Stroke (with hypotension)
Arteriolar and venous vasodilators						
Nitroprusside (Nipride)	0.5–5 min	0.5 μg/kg/min (10 ml/hr) 50 mg in 250 ml of 5% dextrose in water	Every 5 min adjustments 1–3 μg/kg/min (20–40 ml/hr)	10 μg/kg/min (100 ml/hr of double-strength or 50 ml/hr of quadruple strength)	Malignant hypertension With intravenous beta blocker for aortic dissection	Thiocyanate toxicity (Tinnitus, blurred vision, delirium. Keep thiocyanate levels below 10; higher toxicity in renal insufficiency) Cyanide toxicity (Metabolic acidosis, resistance to hypotensive effect, dyspnea, vomiting, dizziness, ataxia; *thiocyanate levels do not correlate with cyanide level*; higher toxicity in hepatic insufficiency. Monitor anion gap and bicarbonate.) Discontinue for tachyphylaxis

Nitroglycerin (venous >> arteriolar)	≤ 5 min	5–10 μg/min (3–6 ml/hr) 25 mg in 250 ml of 5% dextrose in water	5 min	≥ 200 μg/min	Hypertension with coronary ischemia	Avoid in inferior infarction if right ventricular function is impaired Binds to polyvinyl chloride. Need special administration set.
Ganglionic blockers						
Trimethaphan (Arfonad)	—	2 mg/min (60 ml/hr) 500 mg in 250 ml of 5% dextrose in water or normal saline	3–4 mg/min (90–120 ml/hr)	≥ 6 mg/min (180 ml/hr or 90 ml/hr of double-strength)	Aortic dissection	Tachycardia Ileus Dry mouth Angina Urinary retention Pyrosis Cycloplegia Mydriasis Urticaria (releases histamine) Tachyphylaxis
ACE inhibitors						
Enalaprilat (Vasotec IV)	0.25–4 hr	0.625–1.25 mg over 5 min or more	1–6 hr 1.25 mg every 6 hr	20 mg/day	Parenteral maintenance or initiation of therapy	Excessive hypotension if on diuretics or hypovolemic
Magnesium sulfate						
Magnesium sulfate	After loading	*Load:* 5 gm over 10 min *Drip:* 1 gm/hr	0.5–1.5 gm/hr Keep level 6–9 Judge doses clinically by reflexes	—	Toxemia	Paralysis Apnea (toxic doses)

* Doses are average starting doses for a 70-kg patient.

† Also see Appendix X for further information on agents available orally.

REFERENCES

1. Gifford RW (chairman), et al: The fifth report of the Joint National Committee on Detection, Evaluation and Treatment of High Blood Pressure (JNC V). Arch Intern Med 1993;153:154–183.
2. DeVault GA Jr: Therapy in hypertensive emergencies: A disease-specific approach. J Crit Illness 1991;6:477–484.
3. Calhoun DA, Oparil SO: Treatment of hypertensive crisis. N Engl J Med 1990;323:1177–1184.
4. Gifford RW: Management of hypertensive crises. JAMA 1991;266:829–835.

APPENDIX X

Nonparenteral Drugs Used for Treatment of Urgent Hypertension

APPENDIX X

Nonparenteral Drugs Used for Treatment of Urgent Hypertension

Medication	Initial Dose and Followup Dosing	Onset	Duration	Comments
Nifedipine	10 mg capsule crushed and swallowed	5–20 min	3–5 hr	Unpredictable response May cause stroke and myocardial infarction[1,2]
Clonidine[3]	0.2 mg, then 0.1 mg/hr to max of 0.6 mg total dose	30–60 min	6–12 hr	Good for clonidine-withdrawal hypertension
Captopril	6.25–25 mg	15 min	2–6 hr	Risk of hypotension if volume depleted, on diuretics, or have renal artery stenosis

REFERENCES

1. O'Mailia J, Sander GE, Giles TD: Nifedipine-associated myocardial ischemia or infarction in the treatment of hypertensive urgencies. Ann Intern Med 1987;107:185–106.
2. Zeller KR, Von Kuhnert L, Mathews C: Rapid reduction of severe asymptomatic hypertension: A prospective randomized trial. Arch Intern Med 1989;149:2186–2189.
3. Anderson RJ, Hart GR, Crumpler CP, et al: Oral clonidine loading in hypertensive urgencies. JAMA 1981;246:848–850.

INDEX